KW-051-605

MID CLA...
LIBRARY
COLLEGE OF NURSING AND MIDWIFE...

Counselling the coronary patient and partner

David R Thompson
BSc, PhD, RGN, RMN, ONC

Submitted in partial fulfilment of the
requirements for the award of
Doctor of Philosophy from
Loughborough University of Technology

ROYAL COLLEGE OF NURSING
RESEARCH SERIES

Scutari Press

616.12
THO

Aims of the Series
To encourage the appreciation and dissemination of nursing research by making relevant studies of high quality available to the profession at reasonable cost.

The RCN is happy to publish this series of research reports. The projects were chosen by the individual research worker and the findings are those of the researcher and relate to the particular subject in the situation in which it was studied. The RCN in accordance with its policy of promoting research awareness among members of the profession commends this series for study but views expressed do not necessarily reflect RCN policy.

Scutari Press

Viking House, 17–19 Peterborough Road,
Harrow, Middlesex HA1 2AX, England

A subsidiary of Scutari Projects, the publishing company of the Royal College of Nursing

© Scutari Press 1990

All rights reserved. No part of this publication may be reproduced, stored in a retrieval system or transmitted, in any form or by any means, electronic, mechanical, photocopying or otherwise, without the prior permission of Scutari Press, Viking house, 17–19 Peterborough Road, Harrow, Middlesex HA1 2AX, England.

First published 1990

British Library Cataloguing in Publication Data:
Thompson, David R.
   Counselling the coronary patient and partner.
   1. Coronary heart patients. Recovery. Psychological factors
   I. Title   II. Series
   616.1230019

   ISBN 1–871364–42–6

Typeset by Action Typesetting Ltd., Gloucester
Printed and bound in Great Britain by
Billing & Sons, Worcester

26.10.92

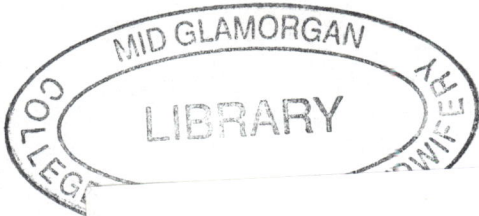

WA 1058130 8

MID GLAMORGAN COLLEGE LIBRARY MIDWIFERY

616.12 THO

BOOK No.........................

Co

STANDARD LOAN
UNIVERSITY OF GLAMORGAN
GLYNTAFF LEARNING RESOURCES CENTRE
Pontypridd, CF37 4BL
Telephone: (01443) 483153
Books are to be returned on or before the last date below

13 JAN 2003

Rt 6 Feb

11 OCT 2004

28 SEP 2004   14 FEB 2005

0 1 NOV 2004   0 6 MAY 2005

13 JAN 2006

0 1 JUN 2006

2 3 OCT 2006

– 5 NOV 2008

2 1 SEP 2007

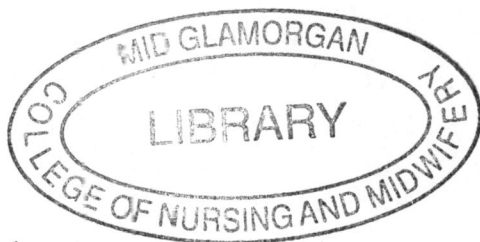

MID GLAMORGAN COLLEGE OF NURSING AND MIDWIFERY LIBRARY

Contents

COLLEGE OF NURSING AND MIDWIFERY LIBRARY

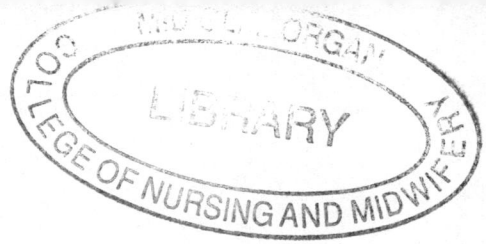

Acknowledgements

Thanks are due to my academic supervisor, Dr Ray Meddis, to Chris Cordle, my clinical colleagues and the patients and spouses who were, and are, the reason for any attempt to better the provision of care.

Thanks are also due to Dr George Pohl for helpful comments and generous financial assistance.

A special debt of gratitude is owed to Rose Webster for her usual selfless help in the data collection and for her support and encouragement when I most needed it.

Part of this work was supported by a Department of Health Nursing Research Studentship, for which I am grateful.

David Thompson

Abstract

The purpose of this study was to monitor and compare levels of anxiety, depression, satisfaction and knowledge in male coronary patients and their spouses throughout the patients' stay in hospital and at 1, 3, and 6 months after discharge from the hospital. A programme of in-hospital educative-supportive counselling was introduced to determine whether or not it significantly affected reactions.

The study design took the form of a randomised controlled trial. The counselling was provided to couples during four 30-minute sessions by a coronary care unit registered nurse.

Findings from the study provide evidence to support the overall contention that this simple programme confers additional benefits over and above the usual management regimen. These benefits include statistically significant reductions in reported anxiety and depression, and increases in satisfaction and knowledge in both partners.

The programme of support was simple and easy to implement, requiring little investment in training personnel and none in additional staff, finances or other resources.

It is concluded that in-hospital counselling for coronary patients and their partners is therapeutically effective and efficient.

Proposals are made for practice change and recommendations are given for the direction of future research.

Dedication

To my son, Luke, in the hope that, in part, it makes up for the time that should have been his.

LIBRARY

COLLEGE OF NURSING AND MIDWIFERY

1 | Psychological reactions to acute myocardial infarction

The experience of suffering a heart attack (myocardial infarction or MI) is virtually always frightening and painful, arousing intense distress in the patient and family, especially the spouse. Later, as the fear of death recedes, they are confronted with the consequences of physical impairment and the experience of surviving a sudden, life-threatening crisis. The patient and spouse, in particular, are likely to be faced with an uncertain future and worry about the patient's ability to resume work, the fulfilment of family obligations and the curtailment of activities that have been important sources of satisfaction and support.

PSYCHOLOGICAL REACTIONS

There is now available an impressive body of evidence confirming that a significant proportion of coronary patients experience at least some degree of emotional distress, which may be denied or suppressed.

According to Hackett and Cassem (1984), the psychological symptoms encountered are mainly centred around two states of mind: anxiety and depression. In a review of the literature, these authors suggest that anxiety

'is a state resembling fear. The sufferer being apprehensive and hyperalert, with signs of heightened autonomic activity' (p.437).

The main reason for the anxiety is the threat of sudden death, although other worries, such as the ability to resume work and leisure activities and to function successfully within the family and society, may be contributory factors.

Hackett and Cassem view depression as

'a state of sadness due to a loss, often of strength, energy, or independence' (p.437).

Other psychological problems experienced during recovery from an acute myocardial infarction, such as insomnia, irritability and loss of libido, usually have their roots in underlying depression. Hackett et al (1968) have reported that this depression is reactive in nature and rarely assumes psychotic proportions. They emphasise that it is a normal response to sustaining a myocardial infarction and is often masked by the patient's fear of death, worry about diagnosis and concern about the immediate future.

Anxiety and depression are often compounded by lack of information, misunderstanding about the heart attack and expected rates of activity and recovery, and inadequate, vague and conflicting advice (Mayou et al, 1976).

The emotional and social responses of patients and their families, particularly spouses, to acute myocardial infarction may be conveniently considered under the following headings:

● Response to hospital.
● Response after discharge.
● Response of the spouse.

Response to hospital

The initial emotional response of patients has been documented by Hackett et al (1968), who conducted a series of 10 studies on 50 myocardial infarction patients in a coronary care unit (CCU). In one study, judgments of predominant mood for each of the patients were made from a variety of sources, including nursing records, observations by relatives, impressions by the investigator and subjective reports from the patient himself. Anxiety was judged to be present when the patient complained of being anxious, when he appeared nervous, sweaty or restless, or constantly requested reassurance or medication. Depression was judged to be present either when the patient appeared despondent and tearful or when he admitted, during interview, to sadness or discouragement. Forty of the 50 patients were judged to be anxious, and 29 admitted being depressed or exhibited behaviour consistent with depression. The majority of patients were either reassured by the cardiac monitor or indifferent to its presence. Dominian and Dobson (1969) studied 74 consecutive male first myocardial infarction patients admitted to a CCU. Only six patients found the unit anxiety-provoking.

The course of emotional changes following acute myocardial infarction was first documented by Cassem and Hackett (1971). Of 441 consecutive patients admitted to a CCU, 145 (32.7%) were referred by a nurse or physician, or both, to the authors for psychiatric consultation. The most frequent reason for referral was anxiety (47 cases), stemming from fear of death or physiological complications, and depression (44 cases), related to decreased self-esteem. Other patients were referred for a variety of management problems, stemming from excessive denial of illness, inappropriate euphoric or sexual behaviour, or hostile conflicts with staff.

Based on the timing and nature of requests for these consultations, Cassem and Hackett developed a model for the time course of such distress. According to the model, anxiety predominates during the first 2 days in a CCU and subsequently declines. This diminished anxiety is a function of the defence mechanism of denial, which is usually predominant on the second day. Depression peaks on the third and fourth days as the impact of the heart attack is felt.

Although this time model was based on experience with only those patients referred to Cassem and Hackett for psychiatric consultation, subsequent reports have tended to confirm and extend the ubiquity and time course for such reactions. For instance, in a series of in-depth studies, Cay and her colleagues (Cay et al, 1972a, b, 1973; Dellipiani et al, 1976; Vetter et al, 1977; Philip et al, 1979) systematically documented and delineated the frequency, type and severity of psychological reactions in coronary patients admitted to hospital. Serial measurements have generally demonstrated that anxiety is highest on admission to the CCU and immediately after transfer to the ward, falling rapidly over the following week and rising just prior to discharge.

Cay et al (1972b) reported psychological disturbances in 62% of the 203 men they studied 8 to 10 days after their first myocardial infarction. The predominant symptoms were anxiety and depression, the assessment being based on clinical interview with no attempt to measure the severity of these symptoms.

Stern et al (1976), also relying on clinical assessment, found 49% of patients to be anxious or depressed during their stay in hospital.

Mayou et al (1978b) rated psychological symptoms on a four-point scale 1 week after admission and found 78% of the first myocardial infarction patients they studied to be mildly or moderately distressed.

Studies that have looked at age of the patient (Billing et al, 1980) and physical severity of the infarct (Cay et al, 1972a, b, 1973; Dellipiani et al, 1976; Stern et al, 1976) have found that these are unrelated to the occurrence of either anxiety or depression, although Vetter et al (1977) found that women patients admitted to a CCU were considerably more anxious than were men.

In a recent study (Silverstone, 1987) of 108 patients admitted consecutively with a diagnosis of myocardial infarction, 48 were classified as depressed as assessed by the Montgomery–Asberg rating scale (Montgomery and Asberg, 1979) between 2 and 24 hours after admission. Of these 48 patients, eight died and six suffered either a cardiac arrest with successful resuscitation or further infarction. Of the 60 who were not depressed, one died and one suffered a further infarction. The author concluded that depression in the first 24 hours after myocardial infarction is an indicator of considerably increased risk of early death, reinfarction or cardiac arrest.

Several studies (Hackett et al, 1968; Klein et al, 1968; Dominian and Dobson, 1969) have noted adverse effects (including anxiety, depression, reinfarction and arrhythmias) associated with transfer from the CCU to general medical wards. In one study, Klein et al (1968) found fewer of these changes among patients who were systematically prepared for transfer and who were each followed throughout and after their hospital stay by a designated nurse and physician.

Response after discharge

The emotional distress, particularly depression, of most coronary patients reaches a peak after discharge from hospital. Wishnie et al (1971) found that of the 24 patients who reported that they were looking forward to returning home, 21 rated themselves as being anxious or depressed 3 to 9 months after discharge. Cay et al (1973) found that over half of the patients they studied remained 'emotionally upset' after 4 and 12 months. This 'emotional upset' (a term used, although not defined, by the authors) seemed to be related to whether or not a person had returned to work.

In two studies of males who had suffered a first heart attack, Thompson et al (1982, 1987) found high levels of anxiety at 6 weeks post-discharge. Specific sources of anxiety reported by these patients included return to work, the future and possible complications.

During the first month following a heart attack, depression is reinforced by a subjective sense of weakness and fatigue. Thereafter, it frequently resolves. However, Stern et al (1976, 1977) found that between 15 and 20% of all post-infarction patients were depressed 1 month after discharge. If left untreated, three-quarters of these continued to be depressed, and half were even more markedly depressed 1 year after infarction.

Response of the spouse

The threat associated with myocardial infarction causes various problems for the whole family, in particular the spouse. The spouse is frequently forgotten in an environment essentially devoted to patient, but not family, care. Yet it is frequently the spouse who has a major role in the patient's readjustment during convalescence and her behaviour is an important determinant of the rate and extent of the patient's recovery.

Cay (1982) has claimed that wives are more anxious than their husbands, at least during the initial period of illness. Certainly, the period following the patient's discharge from hospital is particularly stressful for the wife, who often feels vulnerable, unsupported and overprotective towards her husband.

Wishnie et al (1971) in their interviews with 18 patients and their families 3 to 9 months after the patients' heart attack, found that all of the families demonstrated significant anxiety about the patient's recuperation and their role in promoting or retarding the process. Wishnie et al reported that

'The wives in particular tended to overprotect their husbands in an aggressive way. They felt guilty at having been somehow instrumental in the genesis of the heart attack and were frustrated at being unable to express grievances and anger lest such action bring on another M.I.' (p.1294).

Skelton and Dominian (1973) found that 25 of the 65 wives interviewed 3 months after their husband's myocardial infarction suffered from feelings of anxiety, depression, tension, sleep disturbance, appetite disturbance and (in some) psychosomatic symptoms. Of these 25 wives, 22 experienced severe grief while their husband was in hospital. In two studies (Mayou et al, 1978a, b), 82 wives of men suffering a first myocardial infarction reported considerable distress at 1 week, 2 months and 1 year following their husband's admission to hospital. At 1 year, 18 reported severe 'mental disturbance' and 19 reported moderate 'mental disturbance'.

Apart from high levels of anxiety and depression post-discharge, spouses express dissatisfaction with the quality and quantity of information and support they have received from health professionals. In a series of studies, Mayou and his colleagues found that the spouse as well as the patient had a low level of understanding of advice and information (Mayou et al, 1976), and that the family suffered consequences that were often as great as for the patient (Mayou et al, 1978a, b, c). They drew attention to the important role of the spouse in the patient's readjustment during convalescence and her influence on the rate and extent of the patient's recovery. They concluded that more practical help and advice should be provided for wives of coronary patients during the hospital stay, and for the whole family throughout convalescence.

Hentinen (1983) found that most of the 59 wives she studied reported various signs of stress, particularly insomnia and fatigue, as well as dissatisfaction with professional advice and support. Even when support and information are routinely provided to wives during their husband's stay in hospital, a significant proportion report physical and emotional distress and general dissatisfaction (Thompson and Cordle, 1988).

Apart from feelings of guilt, the spouse may experience various threats, including loss of partner, change in life goals and financial circumstances, a new role within the family and recurrence of myocardial infarction (Bedsworth and Molen, 1982).

In an extensive review of the literature on psychosocial aspects of recovery from ischaemic heart disease, Doehrman (1977) adds information about the strains that arise in the patient's interaction with family members. Fearing another heart attack, they tend to become overprotective or too demanding, and family tensions are common during the recovery process.

EMOTIONAL FACTORS AFFECTING OUTCOME

Several studies suggest that depression in coronary patients may be correlated with poor outcome, as measured by poor vocational adjustment (Nagle et al, 1971; Wishnie et al, 1971; Cay et al, 1973), morbidity and mortality (Garrity and Klein, 1975). For instance, Stern et al (1976) compared with other myocardial infarction patients those who were depressed and found that they had a statistically significantly higher rate of hospital readmission, a decreased ability to remain employed and a greater decrement in sexual functioning.

Cay et al (1973) demonstrated that past coping style, social problems and social class were related to subsequent emotional disturbance and failure to return to work post-MI.

A study by Byrne and Whyte (1978) revealed eight dimensions of illness behaviour that characterised a population of survivors of myocardial infarction. These were clinically identified as:

- somatic concern;
- psychosocial precipitants;
- affective disruption;
- affective inhibition;
- illness recognition;
- subjective tension;
- sick role acceptance;
- trust in the doctor.

Later, these authors (Byrne et al, 1981; Byrne, 1982a) showed that several of these dimensions that were evident 10 to 14 days after the first infarction were predictive of outcome. For example, those patients with poor cardiological outcomes 8 months post-MI were more likely than others to have expressed concern about somatic functioning, and to have recognised the contribution made by life stressors, soon after initial myocardial infarction. Those failing to return to work after 8 months were more likely than others to have accepted the sick role and expressed a subjective feeling of tension following the infarction. However, in a follow-up study, Byrne (1982b) addressed outcome in 73% of the cohort 2 years after infarction. The author concluded that illness behaviour soon after MI related only tenuously to cardiological and occupational outcome after 2 years. This was in contrast with associations evident at 8 months after infarction, suggesting that the most important influences of illness behaviour on outcome occur within the first 8 months after MI.

A number of other reports (Lloyd and Cawley, 1978, 1982, 1983; Philip et al, 1981; Mayou, 1984; Wiklund et al, 1984; Trelawny-Ross and Russell, 1986) have suggested that some premorbid and, more significantly, early post-infarction psychosocial factors are predictive of long-term psychological and social adjustment. These factors include premorbid psychological and social functioning and mental state in hospital.

CONCLUSION

It is clear that patients and their partners experience significant distress during the acute phase of the illness and have considerable difficulties confronting them following discharge. Problems include returning to work, continuing with leisure activities and resuming previous social commitments and responsibilities against a background of fear of possible complications, which remains long after the damaged myocardium has healed.

2 | Acute psychological intervention

It is evident from Chapter 1 that both the patient and family, especially the spouse, experience considerable emotional distress during the acute phase of the patient's illness. This distress, particularly anxiety and depression, tends to peak following discharge from hospital. If steps are not taken to alleviate this, symptoms tend to persist and a year later, half the survivors still have symptoms, which are significantly disturbing in 25% (Cay, 1982). These psychological sequelae of myocardial infarction have a deleterious effect on recovery in terms of morbidity, mortality and resumption of a pre-infarct life-style.

Several major themes emerge from a number of comprehensive reviews of the literature on coronary patient reactions (Croog et al, 1968; Doehrman, 1977; Razin, 1982), some of which have been extrapolated by Razin (1985). For instance:

- There is significant emotional distress, family turmoil and occupational problems in about one quarter of patients at 1 year post-myocardial infarction. However, reports of distress have ranged from 20% (Hinohara, 1970) to 64% (Mayou et al, 1978b) of patients. This discrepancy between studies may be attributed to differences in criteria for psychological distress, populations studied and/or the type and timing of measurements.
- Typical coronary patients do *not* experience short- or long-term emotional disturbances as a result of CCU events and procedures, such as witnessing a cardiac arrest or being connected to a cardiac monitor.
- Occupational adjustment problems are greater among manual workers, less-educated patients, those with lasting

emotional distress and those with more serious medical problems.

- At 1 year post-infarction, about 60% of patients have not returned to previous levels of sexual activity, usually due to reasons such as decrease in sexual desire, depression, anxiety and fear of relapse or sudden death (Hellerstein and Friedman, 1970; Bloch et al, 1975).

- Higher socioeconomic status and marital stability seem to be associated with a good outcome.

- The role of the defence mechanism of denial remains unclear in facilitating or deferring recovery.

- 'Cardiac invalidism' seems to be a common (reported in as many as 50% of patients [Wynn, 1967]), and frequently refractory, problem but may be preventable by appropriate, *early* psychosocial and medical intervention.

Surviving a myocardial infarction is an experience that can have far-reaching consequences for the physical, psychological and social well-being of the patient and family. A multidisciplinary approach to patient management is nowadays well accepted, and a range of therapeutic interventions are available to clinical staff. Some clinicians have placed great reliance on physical conditioning (exercise), whereas others have selected mainly psychological interventions, such as counselling, behaviour therapy and health education.

EXERCISE PROGRAMMES

Exercise training certainly results in numerous physiological benefits for the coronary patient. However, despite improved cardiorespiratory fitness, there is little controlled evidence that it prolongs life or reduces the risk of reinfarction (Blumenthal and Emery, 1988). There is also a paucity of evidence to show that it improves psychosocial functioning. The most comprehensive study has involved 651 male patients who had suffered at least one myocardial infarction, randomly assigned to either an exercise or a control group and assessed with a wide variety of psychosocial measures at the outset and after 6 months, 1 year and 2 years (Stern and Cleary, 1982). However, the investigators failed to find any long-term advantage of exercise on any of the psychosocial variables. Roviaro et al (1984) found that 28 male cardiac patients who participated in a structured exercise programme reported more positive self-perception and better psychosocial functioning than those in a non-randomised control group. However, only 16 of the 28 patients in the treatment group and 12 of the 20 controls had suffered a myocardial infarction. Although exercise programmes generally appear attractive to patients and physicians, they are expensive and require supervision.

Perkins et al (1986), briefly reviewing the contribution of exercise programmes, concluded that the effects of rehabilitation programmes

> 'where physical conditioning is the major component, have been overestimated; they appear to hold little advantage over routine medical follow-up' (p.359).

PSYCHOLOGICAL INTERVENTION

Although the proven efficacy of psychological and educational intervention in other medical and surgical conditions is well documented, there is a relative paucity of such systematic information in coronary patients.

In a comprehensive review of the literature, Blanchard and Miller (1977) suggested that even though psychological intervention has usually only been used as an adjunct to physical conditioning, it would seem to have some advantage over no psychological treatment at all. This was confirmed by Mumford et al (1982), who, in a meta-analysis of 34 controlled, experimental studies, demonstrated that, in general, surgical or coronary patients who are provided with information or emotional support to help them to cope with the crisis have a more favourable outcome than do patients who receive only ordinary care. Although most of the interventions were modest, they offered humane and considerate care, and they can be cost-effective.

Wenger (1982) has emphasised the goal of education and counselling as the provision of information concerning the myocardial infarction and its management, thereby encouraging the patient to become responsible for his or her own state of health. Gottlieb (1983) suggests that

'Supportive interventions can be introduced to foster psychosocial adaptation and adherence to medical regimens. By combining emotional support and patient education, they can induce more benign appraisals of the threats imposed by illness, thus mitigating attendant anxieties, and teach self-care practices' (p.160).

Thus a major function of psychological support is to assist the coronary patient in coping with the traumatic event of his or her illness, reducing the likelihood of chronic anxiety and depression. It is evident that such interventions should be instigated as early as possible.

Based on his extensive review of the literature, Razin (1985) suggests a useful framework on which to base routine post-myocardial infarction intervention:

- Intervention must be early.
- Intervention must be specific, systematic, graduated and educative.
- Specific attention should be paid to depression.
- Social supports must be involved and mobilised.
- Continuity and follow-up are essential.

A number of studies has addressed psychological interventions for coronary patients, including risk factor education and modification, and supportive interventions, whether they be for individuals or groups (Adsett and Bruhn, 1968; Rahe et al, 1973; Ibrahim et al, 1974; Fielding, 1979; Rahe et al, 1979; Horlick et al, 1984; Roviaro et al, 1984). Very occasionally, they have specifically included the spouse (Dracup, 1985). However, these studies exclusively describe care initiated and delivered after the patient has been discharged from hospital. By virtue of the timing of these interventions, they represent not acute psychological intervention but, rather, cardiac rehabilitation. They are, therefore, not the concern of this thesis.

By comparison, the systematic investigation of acute (i.e. in-hospital) psychological intervention in coronary patients has been remarkably limited. Yet, as Perkins et al (1986) suggest, it is probable that the in-hospital phase affords an ideal opportunity to deal with crucial psychosocial issues at a time when the patient and spouse are most aware of them and most likely to be motivated to make any necessary changes. A further advantage is the possibility of intervening with all patients after a myocardial infarction. It would seem sensible to provide the couple with an optimistic, albeit realistic, and informed outlook from the outset, recognising the important contribution of the spouse.

Four studies (Acker, 1976; Cromwell et al, 1977; Naismith et al, 1979; Young et al, 1982), which describe different interventions initiated in hospital, although not exclusively falling within the province of this thesis, merit some attention here.

Interventions initiated in hospital

Acker (1976) compared patients given routine coronary care and hospital rehabilitation with a special care group. The latter were provided with a special patient area, activity and educational schemes, psychological support and a vigorous orientation towards recovery. The average number of days spent in hospital was significantly shorter in the latter group (19.3 *vs* 22.7 days), whose convalescence time was also reduced (78.9 *vs* 100.9 days). The differences in rate of returning to work or re-employment were most marked among the younger (less than 50 years old), lower social class patients.

The patterns observed in this study may have been due to the amount of attention and interest shown in the patients, rather than to specific effects of the procedures themselves. Also, nowadays, the difference in hospital stay is unlikely to be so apparent − the average length of stay is usually between 5 and 10 days.

A highly detailed evaluation of different forms of attention was provided by Cromwell et al (1977) in a comparison of coronary care regimens. They studied 183 patients who were assigned to one of eight psychological treatment groups in a $2 \times 2 \times 2$ factorial design. Three factors were manipulated:

1. *Amount of information:* The *high information* group was given detailed information about the nature and severity of the heart condition and the CCU, together with advice on recovery, diet, work and risk behaviour. The *low information* group was given the conventional description of the CCU and hospital procedures.
2. *Amount of diversion:* The *high diversion* group had television, windows near their beds, reading material and relaxed visiting hours, while these sources were restricted in the *low diversion* group.

3.   *Amount of participation:* The *high participation* group patients
     were encouraged to involve themselves in the recovery
     process. They could switch on their electrocardiographs
     when they experienced symptoms and were given systematic
     exercise schedules in the CCU. By contrast, *low participation*
     group patients were treated with complete bedrest and little
     movement.

Each patient was assigned as 'high' or 'low' on each of
Cromwell et al's factors. Patients allocated to the low information,
low diversion and low participation group were not deprived but
were in the position common in most CCUs at that time. All
patients received the same intensive nursing.

The dependent variables of the intervention study were various
indices of recovery (*vs* recurrence of myocardial infarction and/or
death), comfort and co-operation. Unfortunately, the obvious
differences in treatment format prevented a blind assessment of
recovery, and subtle fluctuations in medical care may have been
present. Nevertheless, although the psychological interventions
showed no appreciable impact upon the long-term indices of
recovery (such as death within 12 weeks or recurrence of acute
myocardial infarction within 12 weeks), a remarkable impact was
shown upon the length of CCU and hospital stay. This stay was
longest among patients who received high information, low
diversion and low participation (mean of 28.0 days), in contrast to
those who received high information and either high levels of
diversion (19.5 days) or participation (20.9 days). Those exposed
to high levels on all three factors recovered at an intermediate rate.

The study suggests that information alone is not sufficient to
promote change. Information is helpful, provided that it is coupled
with some practical action. It also suggests that information
presented during the patient's stay in hospital is assimilated.

Naismith et al (1979) carried out a study in which 68 male
coronary patients aged less than 60 years were counselled on the
third day after infarction by a rehabilitation team consisting of a
physician and nurse. Counselling continued for the next 6
months, when deemed necessary, first in hospital and then at
home. Both patient and spouse were encouraged during these
sessions to speak freely about their activities and difficulties.
These patients were compared to 75 controls who received normal
care following infarction.

At 6 months, the intervention group were deemed more socially independent, and they returned to working life earlier. The rehabilitation was evidently most successful in a sub-sample of 'introverted neurotics'.

Young et al (1982) compared 97 first myocardial infarction patients (male and female) aged less than 66 years, who participated in a rehabilitation programme, with 100 controls. The intervention consisted of the following elements:

- Education about risk factors, ischaemic heart disease, myocardial infarction, expected recovery and medications (provided by a nurse or a health team).
- Education about diet (provided by a dietitian).
- Encouragement of graduated physical activity (provided by a physiotherapist).
- Consultation about work prospects.

Treatment effects were measured at 3 months and 1 year after discharge. When compared with the control group at the 3-month follow-up, treated patients more frequently adhered to recommended diet, lost more weight, were more active, and had lower serum cholesterol levels and less severe angina. However, at the 1-year follow-up, only the difference in cholesterol persisted, thus indicating a decay in the influence of the programme over the observation period and an inability to affect outcomes.

Interventions confined to the hospital

Only three well-controlled studies of in-patient psychological intervention have been reported (Gruen, 1975; Langosch et al, 1982; Oldenburg et al, 1985).

Gruen (1975) investigated the extent to which psychotherapeutic measures initiated during hospital stay have an effect on the recovery process. A group of 70 first myocardial infarction patients aged less than 70 years were randomly assigned to either an intervention or a control group. The intervention (individual psychotherapy) was initiated by a psychologist the day after admission and was conducted six times per week during intensive care and subsequently five times per week. Each intervention lasted, on average, 30 minutes.

Findings indicated that the intervention group required a

shorter intensive care period (6.6 *vs* 7.8 days) and also a shorter overall hospital stay (22.5 *vs* 24.9 days) compared to controls. During the second week of hospital stay, fewer supraventricular arrhythmias, fewer symptoms of fatigue and less depression were observed in patients receiving therapy. In addition, these patients had a more positive social orientation and returned more quickly to a normal level of activity.

The results of this investigation suggest that well-defined psychotherapeutic measures do contribute to an improvement in the patient's ability to manage the trauma of illness.

In a study of 90 male ischaemic heart disease patients, Langosch et al (1982) compared three groups. The first group consisted of 32 patients who participated in stress management training, the second group consisted of 28 patients taking part in relaxation training, and the third group was a control group of 30 patients. The stress management training programme consisted of eight sessions each lasting 1 hour conducted in hospital over a period of 2 weeks. Both treatments emphasised learning to recognise early cues of tension and to engage in coping techniques (such as relaxation, thought stopping and reduction of negative and production of positive self-statements) to reduce arousal. The authors did not state who carried out the intervention.

Patients receiving therapy were less anxious about social exchanges, were less hurried and more patient, and were more convinced that they were capable of managing stress. They were performing better on some psychological and vocational parameters 6 months later, although the range of measures used was limited, making it impossible to assess whether or not there was a similar improvement in physical and life-style functioning.

In a study of 46 first myocardial infarction patients aged less than 70 years, Oldenburg et al (1985) examined the effects of in-hospital counselling, relaxation and education about heart disease and coronary risk behaviour on psychological and physical health. The relaxation and educational components were administered by means of audio-cassette tapes. Two treatment groups were compared with a control group. One treatment group (the counselling group) received counselling, relaxation therapy and education, whereas the other treatment group (the education group) received only the relaxation and educational components. The control group received routine hospital care. A relaxation tape was given to all intervention patients within 48 hours of admission to the hospital, and three education tapes were given on subsequent days. Individual counselling was conducted over at least six, but no more than 10, 45-minute sessions. The first session took place within 48 hours of admission. The two therapists were a psychologist and a psychiatrist. They were not involved in the administration of questionnaires or the collection of data.

Both treatment groups performed significantly better at follow-up (3, 6 and 12 months), compared with the routine care group, on measures of psychological and life-style functioning.

CONCLUSION

The findings from the studies outlined above indicate that in-hospital counselling for coronary patients is beneficial. Although some of the interventions described were initiated in hospital, they were often continued after discharge. Others were not purely psychological interventions but, rather, approaches consisting of varying components, such as physical conditioning.

Other problems that emerge include the lack of information about the patients studied (such as age, sex and social class) and their characteristics (for example, many studies fail to distinguish between first and subsequent infarcts), the type of intervention, the measures used and the outcomes. Thus, replication is often difficult, if not impossible.

3 | Rationale for the present research

Despite the well-documented psychological distress that has been associated with myocardial infarction, there have been few reported systematic studies directed at developing, delivering and evaluating a programme of psychological intervention designed specifically for coronary patients.

METHODOLOGICAL CRITICISM OF PREVIOUS STUDIES

The foregoing literature suggests that although in-hospital counselling for coronary patients is desirable and appears beneficial, there is a need for more rigorously designed and executed studies in order to demonstrate unequivocally the efficacy of such intervention.

Methodological criticisms such as small sample sizes, lack of random assignment to groups and reliance on measures that have not been validated, may be levelled at some of the experimental studies reported earlier. The interventions are often inadequately described, with little importance being attached to distinguishing between concepts such as 'information-giving', 'teaching', 'education', or 'counselling', terms often used interchangeably or loosely (Wilson-Barnett, 1988). In addition, none of the studies described in the preceding chapter used staff members who were involved in the routine care of patients after a myocardial infarction to initiate and continue the intervention. Moreover, there has been no intervention study reported to date that has involved the patient's spouse, despite the known impact of the spouse on the recovery process of the coronary patient.

A decade ago Frank et al (1979) concluded that:

- early post-coronary intervention is desirable;
- spouses or significant others should usually be included;
- therapists need not be physicians;
- supportive-educative and behavioural interventions are likely to be the most effective.

Razin (1985) supported and extended such recommendations and specifically suggested that:

- appropriate, well-timed psychological intervention in the acute phase should be *routinely* offered;
- intervention should be didactic, detailed and repetitive;
- an open, honest approach should be taken, showing compassion, confidence and forthrightness;
- there should be awareness of the relative phasic specificity of patient reactions;
- anxiety should be treated supportively and thus minimised whenever possible.

Yet, no published study to date has incorporated most of these key features in its design. Razin (1985) has noted that there is virtually no systematic study of acute-phase intervention. Referring to his suggestions that intervention should be early, systematic, educative and involve social supports, he states that

> 'while it might be tedious to test these recommendations singly, it would be quite valuable to test a number of them in a "package" or comprehensive design' (p.184).

The aim of this study was to attempt to incorporate such features into the design of a package of support. The author was mindful of the conclusions reached by Steptoe (1981)

> 'Enthusiasm for a treatment does not depend simply on its efficacy, but on a whole constellation of secondary factors, including expense, ease of administration, and professional training requirements' (p.229).

The type of psychological intervention that coronary patients and their spouses are most likely to benefit from would appear to be some form of supportive-educative counselling. Coronary care nurses would be ideally placed to undertake such a function by virtue of their expertise in dealing with such patients and their families, being available on a 24-hour basis and able to give more time on a one-to-one basis to provide practical and relevant support and information. They can also initiate any intervention early and follow this up throughout the patient's stay in hospital.

NOVEL FEATURES OF PRESENT STUDY

Novel features of the design included the following:

- Early initiation of psychological intervention (i.e. within 24 hours of admission to hospital), including appropriate measurement, and early and regular follow-up (i.e. at 1, 3 and 6 months after discharge).
- Inclusion of the patient's spouse.
- Provision of the intervention by a CCU registered nurse.
- Examination of specific sources of anxiety.
- Easy administration of the intervention.

It was envisaged that the provision of such a package of support would be simple, easy to administer and not involve reliance on additional staff, finances or other resources.

4 The study design

AIM OF THE STUDY

The main aim of this research was to monitor and compare levels of anxiety, depression, satisfaction and knowledge reported by first myocardial infarction male patients and their spouses throughout the patients' stay in hospital and at 1, 3 and 6 months after discharge from hospital. An independent variable of a programme of nursing support and education was introduced to determine whether or not it significantly affected reactions.

A further aim was to extend and refine some earlier work by the author (Thompson et al, 1982, 1987; Thompson and Cordle, 1988) examining the specific sources and patterns of anxiety in coronary patients and their spouses.

HYPOTHESES

The following three hypotheses were tested:

1. Patients and spouses receiving the programme of in-hospital supportive-educative counselling will report significantly lower levels of anxiety and depression than will those who do not receive such intervention.
2. Patients and spouses receiving the programme of in-hospital supportive-educative counselling will report significantly higher satisfaction than will those who do not receive such intervention.
3. Patients and spouses receiving the programme of in-hospital supportive-educative counselling will obtain significantly

higher knowledge scores than will those who do not receive such intervention.

SETTING

The study was carried out in the modern, spacious and open-plan designed eight-bedded CCU of a large (1000 beds) teaching hospital.

DESCRIPTION OF CARE

The CCU has a progressive nursing and medical approach to patient care.

The nursing establishment comprised 20 qualified general nurses, 12 of whom were registered (including four charge nurses) and eight enrolled. All of the nurses had an average of 3 (range 2 to 8) years' experience of coronary care nursing, and over one third (eight) had obtained appropriate post-basic qualifications.

A system of 'primary nursing' had been in operation for at least 2 years at the time of the study. Essentially, this method of care ensures that one nurse is primarily responsible and accountable for assessing, planning, delivering and evaluating the nursing care of either one or two patients and their families during their stay in the CCU. There was a shift system of internal rotation in operation. Similar nursing systems of care were operated on each of the three medical wards to which patients were transferred.

One consultant physician was responsible for the routine medical management of patients in the CCU. Patients were examined on a daily basis by either the consultant or a senior registrar, in addition to the CCU house officer and senior house officer.

DESIGN

This randomised controlled trial had a prospective, longitudinal, repeated measures design.

A consecutive series of 60 couples was randomly assigned, in cells of 10, to one of two predetermined groups:

1. *Treatment (intervention) group.* These couples received a systematic programme of supportive-educative counselling from one of two registered nurses, in addition to routine medical, nursing and paramedical care.
2. *Control group.* These couples received the routine medical, nursing and paramedical care normally provided to myocardial infarction patients in hospital, but no other intervention.

The inclusion of an attention-placebo group was considered, but it was decided that there were likely to be ethical objections, and, as Wilson-Barnett (1984) has pointed out, there might have been some difficulty in sustaining an unstructured conversation for the necessary duration (30 minutes) for each intervention and a risk to co-operation from patients if they saw this as a waste of time.

This study design was planned in order to avoid contamination of control subjects by any influence of treatment subjects and also to avoid confusion for patients in the different groups who might be receiving different care at the same time. It also minimised the effect of extraneous variables, which may have been introduced during the period of data collection.

RANDOMISATION

The study design incorporated random assignment to reduce bias in the allocation of individuals to experimental groups. In accordance with the suggestion of Pocock (1983), arrangements for consecutive assignment to groups was prepared by an independent person and based on the use of a table of random numbers. This allows completely unpredictable treatment assignment but does, if necessary, permit reproducibility and checking of the method.

Control (A) and treatment (B) group assignment took place in the following sequence (in cells of 10):

Group:	A	B	A	B	B	A
n:	10	10	10	10	10	10

The design required two researchers, who had separate roles during the experimental phase: one acting as data collector, the other providing the experimental intervention programme. One researcher provided the intervention to the first five of the 10 couples in each treatment group, while the other collected the data. The researchers then exchanged roles for the remaining five couples throughout the study to facilitate comparisons of their effect on data and their efficacy as a support agent. Both researchers were experienced coronary care registered nurses.

The approach and content of the intervention package provided by the two researchers were in close agreement, as determined by an independent assessor (a cardiologist).

Nurses on the CCU and wards were not told the group to which patients were assigned.

Both groups received conventional medical care under one consultant physician on the CCU and under one of three others on one of the three medical wards to which they were transferred.

During the entire phase of the study there was no other hospital or community based form of cardiac rehabilitation taking place.

5 | Patients and methods

SUBJECTS

Patients who met the following inclusion criteria were eligible to participate in the study:

- Male, aged less than 65 years.
- Living with a spouse.
- Having suffered a first myocardial infarction.
- Having a coronary prognostic index (CPI) of less than 10 according to the criteria of Norris et al (1969).
- Primarily English speaking.
- Able and willing to participate.

Acute myocardial infarction was considered present if the patient fulfilled at least two of the following three criteria:

1. Myocardial ischaemic pain of more than 30 minutes' duration.
2. Creatine phosphokinase (CPK) level elevated to more than twice the upper limit of normal.
3. Minnesota code (MC) electrocardiographic evidence for acute infarction (Rose et al, 1982).

Ethical approval was sought and granted by the local health authority ethical committee. Patients and spouses gave their consent to take part in this 'Nursing study monitoring patients' and spouses' reactions to hospital'.

INTERVENTION

The intervention was a structured support and education package for the couple regarding the patient's illness and subsequent recovery (appendix I). It was provided in the form of four sessions of counselling, each of 30 minutes' duration. (Counselling is a term frequently used and variously defined. It is a helping activity concerned with helping an individual to use his or her own coping resources. Thus, counselling may be defined as helping someone to explore a problem, clarify conflicting issues and discover alternative ways of dealing with the problem.) Individual needs of the couple were catered for, thus necessitating a degree of flexibility in the nature and extent of the intervention. However, the majority of the support and education that the couple required was fairly general, and most of the time the programme was similar for each couple.

Essentially, the treatment group received standardised education covering the following areas:

- The nature of the heart attack and subsequent management.
- Primary and secondary coronary risk factors and any necessary strategies for modifying them.
- The impact of the heart attack on sexual functioning and social, work and leisure activities.

Couple counselling was focused on the patient's and spouse's reactions to and feelings towards the heart attack. Thus, it encouraged the ventilation of both positive and negative feelings, interpreting thoughts, feelings and behaviour, offering reassurance and support, encouraging the couple to alter their environment, and helping to resolve immediate problems.

The general principles of the treatment programme were:

1. To reduce uncertainty and fear by providing information about:
- the patient's illness: what it is, how it is managed, the likely outcome and possible prevention of recurrence;
- the staff, equipment, routines and general environment of the CCU and ward;
- the staff's expectations of the patient: rate of recovery and rehabilitation, transfer to the ward and length of stay in hospital.
2. To give the couple an optimistic but realistic outlook regarding recovery, in order to ensure that they anticipated possible physical and emotional reactions to a myocardial infarction. For instance, possible angina, breathlessness and

fatigue might be experienced by the patient after arriving home, while the spouse might experience guilt and tearfulness. The significance of such potential reactions was discussed, emphasising that they did not usually indicate complications or impediment to the healing process.

3. To provide a framework of continuous psychological support by forming a trusting relationship to permit the listening to and answering of questions, impart facts, correct misconceptions and dispel fear-inducing myths, but to limit repetition, contradiction and anecdotal information. Any questions that required medical input were referred to the appropriate physician.

4. To enable partners to reflect on any losses (actual or threatened) and discover positive coping mechanisms to deal with them. Negative reactions, particularly anxiety and depression, were discussed. The couple were reassured that these reactions were common and were invited to discuss any concerns, with a view towards discovering alternative approaches to coping with the problem.

5. To involve the couple, through discussion, in decision-making about aspects of care, for instance, explanations about bedrest and graduated activity so that the couple understood the rationale for these and were thus likely to continue to comply with advice following discharge from hospital.

MEASURES

A series of measures, standardised or designed by the author, was selected for the purposes of this study.

Measurements were obtained by the data collector prior to each stage of the intervention programme, the interviewer being blind to the results obtained.

Data were collected from both groups at the time of acceptance into the trial, and at 24 hours, 48 hours, 72 hours, 5 days, 1 month, 3 months and 6 months after admission to the CCU.

Demographic data

Demographic data included:

- age (years);
- social class;
- duration of stay in hospital.

Age
The ages of each patient and spouse were obtained at the time of entry to the study.

Social class
The social class of each patient was obtained using the Registrar General's classification (Office of Population Censuses and Surveys, 1980). The classification is as follows:

I   Professional occupations.
II   Intermediate occupations (including managerial).
IIIN   Skilled occupations (non-manual).
IIIM   Skilled occupations (manual).
IV   Partly skilled occupations.
V   Unskilled occupations.

Duration of stay
The duration of stay in the CCU and ward of each patient was documented in hours.

Health data

Patient health data included:

- systolic and diastolic blood pressure (mmHg);
- body mass index (weight [kg]/height [m^2]);
- tobacco consumption;
- an assessment of the severity of myocardial infarction using a coronary prognostic index (Norris et al, 1969).

Systolic and diastolic blood pressure
Indirect measurements of systolic and diastolic blood pressure were made by one of the two researchers using a Dinamap 845XT Adult/Pediatric Vital Signs Monitor (Critikon Inc., Tampa, Florida, USA), which provides a digital readout of heart rate and mean systolic and diastolic arterial pressures.

Body mass index

From the baseline measurements of height (m) and weight (kg), the body mass index (BMI) was computed. The normal range is 20.1 to 25.0 for males. A BMI of between 25 and 29 indicates that the individual is overweight, while a BMI that exceeds 30 indicates obesity (Royal College of Physicians of London, 1983).

Tobacco consumption

Each patient was asked whether he smoked and, if so, the number of cigarettes or cigars smoked per day. If a pipe was smoked, tobacco consumption was recorded in ounces per day. The spouses were asked to verify this. In addition, at follow-up, an EC50 Carbon Monoxide Monitor (Bedfont Technical Instruments, London) was used as an unbiased, reliable and non-invasive marker (Jarvis et al, 1986). This compact, portable monitor has been designed specifically for smokers' clinics and medical diagnostic applications to measure carbon monoxide concentrations in a subject's end-expired breath.

Coronary prognostic index

The coronary prognostic index (CPI) developed by Norris et al (1969) provides an unbiased method for the assessment of immediate prognosis in infarction and of new forms of treatment for acute myocardial infarction. The index is constructed from numerical weightings given to six easily measurable factors associated with hospital mortality from acute myocardial infarction:

- Age.
- Electrocardiographic assessment of the position and extent of infarction.
- Systolic blood pressure on admission to hospital.
- Heart size.
- Degree of congestion of the lung fields assessed on a chest X-ray.
- History of previous ischaemia.

A CPI of less than 6 indicates a mild, uncomplicated course, whereas a score of between 6 and 9 indicates a moderately ill patient. A CPI of 10 or more indicates a critically ill patient.

Personality data

Eysenck Personality Questionnaire
In order to obtain data on personality characteristics, especially emotionality, the Eysenck Personality Questionnaire (EPQ; Eysenck and Eysenck, 1975) was used (appendix II). The EPQ is a development of various early personality questionnaires. It differs from the Eysenck Personality Inventory (EPI), which includes measures of neuroticism or emotionality (N) and extroversion–introversion (E), and a 'lie' (L) scale to measure dissimulation, by including an additional scale, psychoticism (P) – an underlying personality trait present to varying degrees in all people, although if it is markedly present, it predisposes to the development of psychiatric abnormalities.

The adult version of the EPQ was used, which comprises 90 items to which respondents place a circle around 'Yes' or 'No'. Instructions are printed in each copy of the EPQ. The questionnaires are scored using the appropriate stencil, one for each of the four dimensions (P, E, N and L) to be measured.

Anxiety and depression

Two instruments for measuring anxiety and depression were used: a standardised instrument, the Hospital Anxiety and Depression scale (Zigmond and Snaith, 1983), and a series of visual analogue scales developed by the researcher.

Hospital Anxiety and Depression scale
The Hospital Anxiety and Depression (HAD) scale (appendix III) is a self-assessment instrument for use by adults, designed to detect the mood disorders of anxiety and depression in non-psychiatric populations. It provides separate measures of anxiety and depression, derived from clinical experience rather than factor analysis.

The scale is brief, readily comprehensible and easily completed. Instructions to the respondent are to complete the scale with regard to how he or she feels at present. The instrument consists of two sets of seven items with four-point response scales. The score ranges on the HAD scale are 'normal' (0 to 7), 'borderline' (8 to 10) and 'morbid' (11 to 21) for each subscale. Its main advantage over many other similar self-assessment questionnaires that measure psychiatric morbidity is that it does not probe the somatic symptoms characteristic of some psychological states that could also be due to the physical disease process. The instrument has been extensively used and has a high degree of specificity and sensitivity (Goldberg, 1985), and a number of reports (Snaith and Taylor, 1985, Aylard et al, 1987; Bramley et al, 1988), including cardiological research (Channer et al, 1985, 1987), attest to its validity.

Visual analogue scales

In an attempt to extend and refine earlier work examining specific sources of anxiety in first myocardial infarction male patients (Thompson et al, 1982, 1987) and their spouses (Thompson and Cordle, 1988), eight visual analogue scales (VASs) were designed for each partner.

VASs provide a means of rapid assessment and have been in use for well over 60 years (Hayes and Patterson, 1921) in the assessment of subjective phenomena; their methodological characteristics have been well described (Aitken, 1969; Bond and Lader, 1974; Maxwell, 1978). The clinical application of VASs has recently been critically reviewed by McCormack et al (1988). These authors conclude that VASs have many additional advantages, such as ease of construction and use and versatility, over other comparable psychological measures. McCormack et al (1988) cite claims by proponents, such as Folstein and Luria (1973) and Rampling and Williams (1977), that VASs are suitable for frequent and repeated use, easily understood by subjects, very sensitive, with a discriminating capacity superior to other scales, and allow the use of numerical values suitable for statistical analysis.

Although various presentations are available, it was decided to construct VASs with the following characteristics:

- A graphic scale.
- A length of 10 cm.
- As a continuous line.
- End anchor points.
- Horizontal direction.

It was an important consideration that one scale should measure one dimension. Each VAS was reproduced on a separate sheet of paper with random reversal of end-point categories to avoid position response set. The unipolar scales had anchors 'Not at all anxious' and 'Extremely anxious'. Each patient and spouse was asked to indicate 'How anxious are you about. . .?' by placing a cross at a point on the line for each item that corresponded with the degree of anxiety they were experiencing at the time of completion of the scale.

The patient anxiety VAS (appendix IV) concerned eight factors in the following sequence:

1. General health.
2. Ability to work.
3. Another heart attack.
4. Relations with spouse.
5. Possible complications.
6. Sexual activity.
7. Leisure activity.
8. The future.

The spouse anxiety VAS (appendix V) concerned eight factors in the following sequence:

1. Leisure activity.
2. The future.
3. Sexual activity.
4. General health.
5. Relations with patient.
6. Ability of patient to work.
7. Another heart attack for patient.
8. Possible complications for patient.

Following the recommendation of Aitken (1969), subject responses were scored on the 10 cm line at the intersection of the cross, to the nearest millimetre, producing a 100—point scale. Thus, the VASs were designed to yield scores of one to 100.

Satisfaction

In an attempt to measure patients' and spouses' levels of satisfaction with various aspects of care they received, a series of VASs was constructed.

Using visual analogue scales in the manner described above, patients and spouses were each asked to rate their level of satisfaction on a number of variables. Anchor points were 'Not at all satisfied' and 'Extremely satisfied'. The respondent was asked to indicate 'How satisfied are you with ...?'.

The patient satisfaction VAS (appendix VI) concerned four factors in the following sequence:

1. General health.
2. Life in general.
3. Care received.
4. Information received.

The spouse satisfaction VAS (appendix VII) concerned two factors in the following order:

1. Information received.
2. Care patient received.

Knowledge

In order to evaluate the level of knowledge each patient and spouse had acquired about a myocardial infarction, a simple eight-item questionnaire (appendix VIII) was constructed, which was designed to elicit information about the heart attack, coronary care and convalescent care.

Patients and spouses were each asked to complete the instrument, which consisted of four multiple-choice questions (each comprising four statements to which the response was 'True' or 'False'), two true or false questions and two open-ended questions. The maximum score achievable was 12.

Activity

In order to obtain some indication of the level of general activity each patient was attaining following discharge from the hospital, a VAS was constructed (Appendix IX).

Each patient was asked to compare his present level of activity with his level prior to the heart attack. The end anchor points were 'Definitely worse' and 'Definitely better'. Scores ranged from one ('Definitely worse') to 100 ('Definitely better').

Physical state

Each couple was asked to keep a diary of the frequency, duration and severity of any attacks of angina or shortness of breath (dyspnoea) following discharge from hospital.

Based on these records, each attack was graded as follows:

0   Nil.
1   On moderate/severe exertion.
2   On mild exertion.
3   At rest.

Other Measures

In addition to the measures described, it was decided that the following data regarding patient outcome would be of interest:

- Date of return to work.
- Morbidity (including reinfarction).
- Mortality.
- Readmission to hospital.

ADMINISTRATION OF INSTRUMENTS

Careful consideration was given to the ease and timing of administration of the instruments used. For example, the EPQ is a relatively lengthy instrument that requires a good degree of concentration and takes about 10 to 15 minutes to complete. Therefore, it was felt that it would be most appropriate to administer this on one occasion, about 48 hours after admission. On the other hand, the battery of visual analogue scales for anxiety is easy and quick to complete and, as such, it was felt that this could be administered on each occasion.

A summary of the timing of each measurement is presented in table 1.

PROCEDURE

All patients were admitted directly to the CCU at the request of the general practitioner or ambulance service.

Approximately 24 hours after admission, each couple, who had already been randomly allocated to one of the two groups of the study, was approached by one of the researchers acting as data collector.

The researcher provided a detailed explanation of the study to the couple and then issued an invitation to participate in it.

Table 1 Summary of type and time of measures obtained from study groups

Measure	T1	T2	T3	T4	T5	T6	T7
Hospital Anxiety and Depression Scale:							
Patient and spouse	+			+	+	+	+
Anxiety visual analogue scales:							
Patient and spouse	+	+	+	+	+	+	+
Satisfaction visual analogue scales:							
Patient and spouse		+		+	+	+	+
Knowledge questionnaire:							
Patient and spouse	+			+	+	+	+
Activity scale:							
Patient		+			+	+	+
Eysenck Personality Questionnaire:							
Patient and spouse		+					
Blood pressure:							
Patient	+			+			+
Body mass index:							
Patient	+					+	+

T1 = 24 hours; T2 = 48 hours; T3 = 72 hours; T4 = 5 days; T5 = 1 month; T6 = 3 months; T7 = 6 months.

Provided partners gave their consent, and the patient was pain-free and able, they were each asked to complete a battery of scales. The couple was informed that the questionnaires were being issued for research purposes, and they were reassured that their responses would be confidential and that their care and management would in no way be adversely affected. The couples were not told that they would be given the same questionnaires at later intervals, including at post-discharge follow-up. Neither was there any mention made of the intervention programme being evaluated, and the researchers (data collector and therapist) were careful not to interact, so that couples would not be aware of any formal link between the intervention programme and the evaluation.

The researchers, both experienced registered nurses (one a female staff nurse, the other a male charge nurse, both aged less than 30 years) working on the CCU, wore uniforms and name badges. They introduced themselves by their Christian names and professional status, in accordance with routine practice.

Treatment group

Following data collection by the first researcher, the second researcher (blind to the data) provided the programme of support and information to the treatment group. Each couple was seen for an average of 30 minutes on four occasions: 24 hours, 48 hours, 72 hours and 5 days after admission. The same researcher provided the treatment package for the four occasions, while the other researcher acted as data collector. This was planned in order to ensure that there was a satisfactory degree of continuity.

The first intervention (after 24 hours) in the CCU took place at the patient's bedside. At this early stage, the patient was either in bed or sitting in a reclining chair, with the spouse and researcher sitting nearby. The treatment was generally provided out of earshot of adjacent patients with the curtains drawn, ensuring as much privacy as was practically possible. The second intervention (48 hours), in the CCU, generally took place with the patient sitting at the bedside, whereas on the third (72 hours) and fourth (5 days) occasions, on the ward, the patient was usually ambulant and the interviews took place in more privacy.

At each session the patient and spouse were initially seen together for the bulk of the intervention (lasting about 25 minutes), then later separately (for about 5 to 10 minutes). The spouse was invited into the CCU office by the researcher to provide an opportunity to discuss any pertinent personal problems or issues. When the spouse had left the CCU, the researcher presented the patient with the same opportunity.

Prior to each intervention, the researcher ascertained the couple's level of understanding and activity. This knowledge was reinforced where necessary and the opportunity taken to clarify issues and correct any misconceptions. Each intervention was essentially verbal in content, although both treatment and control groups routinely received a fairly detailed education booklet – *Counter Attack the Heart Attack* (Stuart Pharmaceuticals Ltd., Cheadle) – covering myocardial infarction, coronary care and convalescent care. Each session ended with an opportunity for the couple to discuss any particular concerns that they had.

All couples completed a battery of questionnaires mailed to them at 1 and 3 months after discharge home. Finally, they attended the CCU 6 months post-discharge for an interview with the researcher.

Following discharge from the hospital, all couples were asked to record, in a patient diary, the date, time, severity and duration of any episodes of chest pain.

The researcher acting as therapist was not involved at any stage in the administration of questionnaires or the collection of data, either in the hospital or at any of the follow-up meetings.

PILOT STUDY

Although the researcher had carried out previous work similar to the present study, it was felt necessary that a pilot study should be carried out to assess the feasibility of the research design and evaluate the measuring instruments.

The study design was pilot-tested with five couples who met the entry criteria. The procedure followed the format described above.

The subjects completed the questionnaires without any apparent problems. However, three couples felt that the EPQ was quite a lengthy instrument to complete at 24 hours after admission (the time originally chosen for completion), and it was decided, therefore, that 48 hours might be a more appropriate time.

The intervention did not seem to present any problems to the staff or research subjects, and no refinements were deemed necessary.

The pilot sample was not included in the main study.

STATISTICAL ANALYSIS

Raw scores for all subjects were computed and statistical analysis was performed by one-way analysis of variance (ANOVA) using the MINITAB statistics package (Minitab Inc., Pennsylvania, USA), run on the Honeywell Multics computer system at the University of Technology, Loughborough.

Where appropriate, other statistical analyses were performed using the OMNIBUS system (Meddis, 1984), a BASIC programme run on a BBC Model B computer.

Data were expressed in means and standard deviations where appropriate. Data were considered to be statistically significant at the 0.05 level.

CONFIDENCE INTERVALS

Recently, in the medical and cardiological literature, there have been claims that undue emphasis has been placed on hypothesis testing, detracting from more informative statistical approaches, such as estimation and confidence intervals (Gardner and Altman, 1986; Bulpitt, 1987; Evans et al, 1988). For example, p values convey no information about the sizes of the differences between study groups. The confidence interval, however, provides a range of values that are considered to be plausible for the population.

Where appropriate, the 95% confidence interval (CI) for the difference in means was calculated in addition to p values.

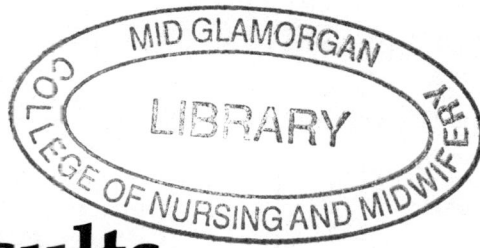

MID GLAMORGAN
COLLEGE OF NURSING AND MIDWIFERY
LIBRARY

6 | Results

Data collection commenced at the beginning of January 1986 and was completed at the end of December 1986. During that period, there were 1034 admissions to the CCU, of whom 386 had suffered an acute myocardial infarction. Two hundred and thirteen were male patients with a first myocardial infarction, but 71 were aged 66 years or more. Of the 142 remaining, 78 were excluded on the basis of a coronary prognostic index (Norris et al, 1969) of 10 or more (37), language difficulties (32) or collapsed state (9). Thus, only 64 patients satisfied the entry criteria. However, by mid-December 60 couples had agreed to participate, and recruitment ceased. Of all those approached, no patients or spouses refused to participate in the study.

No deaths occurred early in the study and no replacements were used. However, after discharge home there were three patient deaths: two in the control group (one occurring within 1 month and the other within 2 months of discharge from the hospital) and one in the treatment group (occurring within 1 month of discharge).

DEMOGRAPHIC AND HEALTH DATA

Baseline demographic and health data of the patient study groups are shown in table 2. A two-tailed test indicated that the differences between groups with respect to patient and spouse age, patient blood pressure, body mass index and peak cardiac enzyme (creatine phosphokinase) level were not statistically significant, suggesting that they were homogeneous with respect to baseline characteristics.

Table 2 Baseline demographic and health data of the study groups

Variable	Treatment (n = 30)		Control (n = 30)		Difference between means	95% confidence interval	F	d.f.	p
	Mean	**S.D.**	**Mean**	**S.D**					
Age (years):									
Patient	52.8	7.4	55.9	7.2	3.1	−0.7 to 6.9	2.67	1,58	n.s.
Spouse	50.4	8.2	54.6	8.3	4.2	0.0 to 8.4	3.50	1,58	n.s.
Blood pressure (mmHg):									
Systolic	137.1	24.1	137.3	22.2	0.2	−11.8 to 12.2	0.00	1,58	n.s
Diastolic	90.9	19.4	89.4	15.4	−1.5	−10.5 to 7.5	0.11	1,58	n.s
Body mass index (kg/m^2)	25.7	2.4	25.8	2.8	0.1	−1.2 to 1.4	0.01	1,58	n.s.
Peak creatine phosphokinase (iu/l)	1500	1359	1459	1205	−41	−703 to 621	0.01	1,58	n.s.

Table 3 shows the social classes of the patient groups. The groups appeared evenly matched with respect to social class, the majority of patients having skilled or partly skilled occupations (social classes III or IV).

Table 3 Social class of the study groups

Social class*	Treatment (n = 30)		Control (n = 30)	
I	1	(3.3%)	1	(3.3%)
II	6	(20.0%)	5	(16.6%)
IIIN	6	(20.0%)	7	(23.3%)
IIIM	4	(13.3%)	3	(10.0%)
IV	10	(33.3%)	10	(33.3%)
V	3	(10.0%)	4	(13.3%)

*Registrar General's classification (Office of Populations Censuses and Surveys, 1980)

Baseline cardiological data, which comprise location and severity of myocardial infarction (according to the coronary prognostic index [CPI] of Norris et al, 1969), are shown in table 4. Each group had an equal proportion of patients who had sustained an anteriorly or inferiorly located infarct. According to the CPI criteria of Norris et al (1969), three-quarters of each patient group were classed as having suffered 'mild, uncomplicated' infarcts, the remainder being classed as moderately ill. It can be seen that there were no critically ill patients (i.e. those with a CPI of more than 9), as these were excluded by the study entry criteria.

Table 4 Location and severity of myocardial infarction in the study groups

Variable	Treatment (n = 30)		Control (n = 30)	
Location:				
Anterior	12	(40.0%)	15	(50.0%)
Inferior	18	(60.0%)	15	(50.0%)
Severity*:				
<6	23	(76.7%)	22	(73.3%)
6−9	7	(23.3%)	8	(26.7%)

*Coronary prognostic index (Norris et al, 1969)

Duration of CCU and ward stay of the study groups is shown in table 5. The average length of stay in the CCU was about 70 hours and on the ward about 102 hours. Thus, the average total duration of stay in the hospital was approximately 1 week.

PERSONALITY CHARACTERISTICS

Eysenck Personality Questionnaire scores
Table 6 shows the mean Eysenck Personality Questionnaire (EPQ) scores for both groups of patients and spouses. There were no statistically significant differences between the groups with respect to the psychoticism (P), extroversion–introversion (E), neuroticism (N) or 'lie' (L) scales.

Although the spouse neuroticism and 'lie' scale scores were higher than those of the patients, these differences are, in fact, a typical reflection of the EPQ norms (Eysenck and Eysenck, 1975).

ANXIETY AND DEPRESSION SCORES

Tables 7 to 10 show the mean Hospital Anxiety and Depression scale scores for both groups. Tables 11 to 26 show the mean visual analogue scale anxiety scores for both groups.

Hospital Anxiety and Depression scale
Patient anxiety.   Table 7 shows the mean anxiety scores for both groups of patients on the five occasions of testing. A one-tailed test revealed that the difference between the baseline (24 hour) scores, which reflect borderline anxiety (Zigmond and Snaith, 1983), were not statistically significant. However, at 5 days there was a dramatic reduction in the mean score of the treatment group compared to the controls, which was significantly different. This trend was maintained at 1, 3 and 6 months.
Patient depression.   Table 8 shows the mean depression scores for both groups of patients on the five occasions. The baseline (24 hour) scores, which reflect a normal range of values, were not statistically significantly different. However, at 5 days and up to 3 months after infarction, a one-tailed test revealed that the scores were significantly lower in the treatment group. At 6 months, the differences were not significant.

Table 5 Duration of hospital stay of the study groups

Variable	Treatment (n = 30)		Control (n = 30)		Difference between means	95% confidence interval	F	d.f.	p
	Mean	S.D.	Mean	S.D.					
CCU stay (hours)	71.2	32.9	68.2	37.1	−3.0	−21.1 to 15.1	0.11	1,58	n.s.
Ward stay (hours)	103.3	31.3	101.1	49.4	−2.2	−23.6 to 19.2	0.04	1,58	n.s.
Total stay (hours)	174.5	49.9	169.4	58.8	−5.2	−33.3 to 23.1	0.13	1,58	n.s.

Table 6 Patient and spouse Eysenck Personality Questionnaire mean scores

Variable	Treatment (n = 30)		Control (n = 30)		Difference between means	95% confidence interval	F	d.f.	p
	Mean	S.D.	Mean	S.D.					
Patient:									
Psychoticism (P)	2.6	2.5	3.3	1.8	0.7	−0.4 to 1.8	1.57	1,58	n.s.
Extroversion–introversion (E)	11.9	4.6	12.2	4.9	1.3	−1.0 to 3.6	0.05	1,58	n.s.
Neuroticism (N)	8.6	5.4	10.6	5.0	2.0	−0.7 to 4.7	2.27	1,58	n.s.
'Lie' (L)	9.3	4.4	8.9	4.4	−0.4	−2.7 to 1.9	0.14	1,58	n.s.
Spouse:									
Psychoticism (P)	1.5	1.5	2.3	2.0	0.8	−0.1 to 1.7	3.44	1,58	n.s.
Extroversion–introversion (E)	10.0	4.4	11.8	4.7	1.8	−0.6 to 4.2	2.26	1,58	n.s.
Neuroticism (N)	11.8	5.3	12.0	6.2	0.2	−2.8 to 3.2	0.01	1,58	n.s.
'Lie' (L)	11.2	4.1	12.8	3.8	1.6	−0.4 to 3.6	2.23	1,58	n.s.

Spouse anxiety. Table 9 shows the mean anxiety scores for both groups of spouses on the five occasions. The baseline (24 hour) scores, which reflect borderline morbid anxiety, were not statistically significantly different. However, on each of the following occasions, a one-tailed test revealed that the scores were significantly lower in the treatment group.

Spouse depression. Table 10 shows the mean depression scores for both groups of spouses on the five occasions. The baseline (24 hour) scores reflect a normal range of values. A one-tailed test revealed that there were no statistically significant differences between the groups on any of the five occasions.

Visual analogue scales

Tables 11 to 18 show the mean visual analogue scale anxiety scores for both groups of patients, while tables 19 to 26 show the scores for both groups of spouses.

Respondents were asked to indicate how anxious they were about the following factors. Scores ranged from one (not at all anxious) to 100 (extremely anxious).

Patient anxiety: general health. Table 11 shows the mean anxiety scores for both groups of patients on the seven occasions. A one-tailed test revealed that the difference between the groups at baseline (24 hours) was not statistically significant. The scores declined in both groups over the seven occasions, but were only significantly lower in the treatment group at 72 hours, 5 days and 6 months.

Patient anxiety: ability to work. Table 12 shows the mean anxiety scores for both groups of patients on the seven occasions. A one-tailed test revealed that the difference between the groups at baseline (24 hours) was not statistically significant. The scores declined on each subsequent occasion in the treatment group but were only significantly lower than the control group at 5 days, 3 and 6 months.

Patient anxiety: another heart attack. Table 13 shows the mean anxiety scores for both groups of patients on the seven occasions. A one-tailed test revealed that the difference between the groups at baseline (24 hours) was not statistically significant. However,

Table 7 Patient Hospital Anxiety and Depression scale mean anxiety scores

Time	Treatment			Control			Difference between means	95% confidence interval	F	d.f.	p
	n	Mean	S.D.	n	Mean	S.D.					
24 hours	30	8.5	4.2	30	8.9	3.9	0.4	−1.7 to 2.5	0.12	1,58	n.s.
5 days	30	4.9	2.8	30	8.7	3.9	3.8	2.0 to 5.6	18.25	1,58	<0.001
1 month	29	4.3	3.0	29	7.5	4.2	3.2	1.3 to 5.1	11.05	1,56	<0.001
3 months	29	4.1	3.1	28	6.5	3.3	2.4	0.7 to 3.1	7.66	1,55	<0.01
6 months	29	4.1	2.9	28	6.0	3.3	1.9	0.3 to 3.5	5.34	1,55	<0.05

Table 8 Patient Hospital Anxiety and Depression scale mean depression scores

Time	Treatment			Control			Difference between means	95% confidence interval	F	d.f.	p
	n	Mean	S.D.	n	Mean	S.D.					
24 hours	30	5.3	3.3	30	5.3	3.3	0.0	−1.7 to 1.7	0.00	1,58	n.s.
5 days	30	3.2	2.5	30	5.3	4.2	2.1	0.3 to 3.9	5.91	1,58	<0.01
1 month	29	3.3	2.1	29	5.0	4.3	1.7	−0.1 to 3.5	3.51	1,56	<0.05
3 months	29	3.1	2.3	28	4.7	3.5	1.6	0.1 to 3.1	4.38	1,55	<0.05
6 months	29	3.1	2.2	28	4.3	3.5	1.2	−0.3 to 2.7	2.39	1,55	n.s.

Table 9 Spouse Hospital Anxiety and Depression scale mean anxiety scores

Time	Treatment			Control			Difference between means	95% confidence interval	F	d.f.	p
	n	Mean	S.D.	n	Mean	S.D.					
24 hours	30	10.9	3.9	30	10.0	4.4	-0.9	-3.0 to 1.2	0.70	1,58	n.s.
5 days	30	7.5	3.3	30	10.2	4.8	2.7	0.6 to 4.8	6.11	1,58	<0.01
1 month	29	7.0	3.9	29	9.0	5.1	2.0	-0.4 to 4.4	3.02	1,56	<0.05
3 months	29	6.3	3.6	28	8.5	4.5	2.2	0.0 to 4.4	3.97	1,55	<0.05
6 months	29	6.1	3.5	28	8.1	4.2	2.0	0.0 to 4.0	4.12	1,55	<0.05

Table 10 Spouse Hospital Anxiety and Depression scale mean depression scores

Time	Treatment			Control			Difference between means	95% confidence interval	F	d.f	p
	n	Mean	S.D.	n	Mean	S.D.					
24 hours	30	6.0	4.2	30	5.2	2.9	-0.8	-2.7 to 1.1	0.73	1,58	n.s.
5 days	30	5.1	3.7	30	5.3	3.6	0.2	-1.7 to 2.1	0.05	1,58	n.s.
1 month	29	4.2	3.1	29	5.2	3.6	1.0	-0.7 to 2.7	1.31	1,56	n.s.
3 months	29	4.0	3.1	28	4.7	3.1	0.7	-0.9 to 2.3	0.68	1,55	n.s.
6 months	29	3.7	2.9	28	4.4	2.8	0.7	-0.8 to 2.2	0.86	1,55	n.s.

Table 11 Patient visual analogue scale mean anxiety scores: general health

Time	Treatment			Control			Difference between means	95% confidence interval	F	d.f.	p
	n	Mean	S.D.	n	Mean	S.D.					
24 Hours	30	51.4	30.6	30	50.3	31.7	-1.1	-17.2 to 15.0	0.02	1,58	n.s.
48 hours	30	38.3	27.1	30	47.4	29.9	9.1	-5.6 to 23.8	1.54	1,58	n.s.
72 hours	30	35.9	27.1	30	48.1	28.7	12.2	-2.2 to 26.6	2.84	1,58	<0.05
5 days	30	29.2	24.0	30	47.9	28.8	18.7	5.0 to 32.4	7.49	1,58	<0.01
1 month	29	30.8	25.0	29	39.5	29.4	8.7	-5.6 to 23.0	1.51	1,56	n.s.
3 months	29	30.1	23.0	28	33.5	22.7	3.4	-8.7 to 15.5	0.31	1,55	n.s.
6 months	29	23.3	17.7	28	36.6	25.6	13.3	1.7 to 24.9	5.24	1,55	<0.05

Table 12 Patient visual analogue scale mean anxiety scores: ability to work

Time	Treatment			Control			Difference between means	95% confidence interval	F	d.f.	p
	n	Mean	S.D.	n	Mean	S.D.					
24 hours	30	47.4	31.6	30	48.4	34.4	1.0	-16.1 to 18.1	0.01	1,58	n.s.
48 hours	30	37.3	28.3	30	44.3	34.2	7.0	-9.2 to 23.2	0.74	1,58	n.s.
72 hours	30	36.1	30.0	30	49.2	32.5	13.1	-3.1 to 29.3	2.60	1,58	n.s.
5 days	30	29.2	26.4	30	45.0	31.3	15.8	0.9 to 30.7	4.47	1,58	<0.05
1 month	29	27.4	24.7	29	36.8	32.2	9.4	-5.7 to 24.5	1.55	1,56	n.s.
3 months	29	25.0	23.8	28	37.0	26.6	12.0	-1.4 to 25.4	3.24	1,55	<0.05
6 months	29	17.9	15.9	28	36.7	29.7	18.8	6.2 to 31.4	9.01	1,55	<0.01

there was a significant reduction in anxiety in the treatment group compared to controls following discharge from hospital (at 1, 3 and 6 months).

Patient anxiety: relations with spouse.   Table 14 shows the mean anxiety scores for both groups of patients on the seven occasions. A one-tailed test revealed that the difference between the groups at baseline (24 hours) was not statistically significant. However, there was a significant reduction for the treatment group compared to the control group at the 3 and 6 month follow-ups.

Patient anxiety: possible complications.   Table 15 shows the mean anxiety scores for both groups of patients on the seven occasions. A one-tailed test revealed that the difference between the groups at baseline (24 hours) was not statistically significant. However, there was a significant reduction for the treatment group compared to controls at 5 days and 1 month post-infarction.

Patient anxiety: sexual activity.   Table 16 shows the mean anxiety scores for both groups of patients on the seven occasions. A one-tailed test revealed that there were no statistically significant differences between groups on any of the seven occasions.

Patient anxiety: leisure activity.   Table 17 shows the mean anxiety scores for both groups of patients on the seven occasions. A one-tailed test revealed that the difference between the groups at baseline (24 hours) was not statistically significant. However, there was a significant reduction in anxiety in the treatment group compared to controls at 5 days and 1, 3 and 6 months.

Patient anxiety: the future.   Table 18 shows the mean anxiety scores for both groups of patients on the seven occasions. A one-tailed test revealed that the difference between the groups at baseline (24 hours) was not statistically significant. However, there was a significant reduction in anxiety in the treatment group compared to controls at 72 hours, 5 days and 1 month.

Spouse anxiety: leisure activity.   Table 19 shows the mean anxiety scores for both groups of spouses on the seven occasions. A one-tailed test revealed that the difference between the groups at baseline (24 hours) was not statistically significant. However,

Table 13 Patient visual analogue scale mean anxiety scores: another heart attack

Time	Treatment			Control			Difference between means	95% confidence interval	F	d.f.	p
	n	Mean	S.D.	n	Mean	S.D.					
24 hours	30	64.0	26.9	30	62.5	34.0	−1.5	−17.3 to 14.3	0.03	1,58	n.s.
48 hours	30	54.0	27.7	30	60.1	30.9	6.1	−9.0 to 21.2	0.65	1,58	n.s.
72 hours	30	51.0	27.6	30	60.2	31.0	9.2	−5.9 to 24.3	1.46	1,58	n.s.
5 days	30	44.4	29.4	30	55.3	27.5	10.9	−3.8 to 25.6	2.20	1,58	n.s.
1 month	29	34.8	24.9	29	49.7	26.4	14.9	1.4 to 28.4	4.87	1,56	<0.05
3 months	29	28.5	20.7	28	42.4	28.8	13.9	0.6 to 27.2	4.36	1,55	<0.05
6 months	29	26.9	20.8	28	43.4	25.6	16.5	4.2 to 28.8	7.10	1,55	<0.01

Table 14 Patient visual analogue scale mean anxiety scores: relations with spouse

Time	Treatment			Control			Difference between means	95% confidence interval	F	d.f.	p
	n	Mean	S.D.	n	Mean	S.D.					
24 hours	30	36.1	28.3	30	34.7	30.4	−1.4	−16.5 to 13.7	0.03	1,58	n.s.
48 hours	30	31.3	26.8	30	29.7	26.6	−1.6	−15.4 to 12.2	0.05	1,58	n.s.
72 hours	30	22.1	20.6	30	27.1	26.2	5.0	−7.1 to 17.3	0.70	1,58	n.s.
5 days	10	22.8	21.4	30	28.2	25.7	5.4	−6.8 to 17.6	0.78	1,58	n.s.
1 month	29	17.6	21.3	29	21.4	20.9	3.8	−7.3 to 14.9	0.48	1,56	n.s.
3 months	29	13.0	15.9	28	22.3	20.9	9.3	−0.5 to 19.1	3.59	1,55	<0.05
6 months	29	14.0	14.2	28	25.6	23.6	11.6	1.3 to 21.9	5.12	1,55	<0.05

Table 15 Patient visual analogue scale mean anxiety scores: possible complications

Time	Treatment			Control			Difference between means	95% confidence interval	F	d.f.	p
	n	Mean	S.D.	n	Mean	S.D.					
24 hours	30	45.4	25.7	30	43.8	30.6	−1.6	−16.2 to 13.0	0.05	1,58	n.s.
48 hours	30	38.2	21.9	30	43.3	24.5	5.1	−6.9 to 17.1	0.71	1,58	n.s.
72 hours	30	37.5	23.8	30	46.3	25.4	8.8	−3.9 to 21.5	1.93	1,58	n.s.
5 days	30	28.5	19.7	30	48.6	27.0	20.1	7.9 to 32.3	10.91	1,58	<0.001
1 month	29	26.5	20.1	29	41.1	26.4	14.6	2.3 to 26.9	5.57	1,56	<0.05
3 months	28	26.0	19.4	28	32.7	23.5	6.7	−4.7 to 18.1	1.36	1,55	n.s.
6 months	28	24.8	19.6	28	33.5	21.3	8.7	−2.1 to 19.5	2.59	1,55	n.s.

Table 16 Patient visual analogue scale mean anxiety scores: sexual activity

Time	Treatment			Control			Difference between means	95% confidence interval	F	d.f.	p
	n	Mean	S.D.	n	Mean	S.D.					
24 hours	30	34.0	28.8	30	33.0	30.5	−1.0	−16.3 to 14.3	0.02	1,58	n.s.
48 hours	30	30.2	26.9	30	26.9	21.7	−3.3	−15.9 to 9.3	0.27	1,58	n.s.
72 hours	30	24.7	26.4	30	24.6	20.7	−0.1	−12.3 to 12.1	0.00	1,58	n.s.
5 days	30	18.8	20.6	30	26.0	23.2	7.2	−4.1 to 18.5	1.60	1,58	n.s.
1 month	29	18.2	25.4	29	21.0	20.2	2.8	−9.3 to 14.9	0.22	1,56	n.s.
3 months	29	15.5	21.3	28	21.4	22.4	5.9	−5.7 to 17.5	1.02	1,55	n.s.
6 months	29	15.3	17.5	28	24.2	23.9	8.9	−2.2 to 20.0	2.59	1,55	n.s.

Table 17 Patient visual analogue scale mean anxiety scores: leisure activity

Time	Treatment			Control			Difference between means	95% confidence interval	F	d.f.	p
	n	Mean	S.D.	n	Mean	S.D.					
24 hours	30	38.9	28.0	30	38.0	31.2	−0.9	−16.2 to 14.4	0.01	1,58	n.s.
48 hours	30	28.7	22.1	30	40.7	32.9	12.0	−2.5 to 26.5	2.74	1,58	n.s.
72 hours	30	25.6	20.1	30	33.9	27.3	8.3	−4.1 to 20.7	1.77	1,58	n.s.
5 days	30	25.1	18.7	30	36.7	24.3	11.6	−0.4 to 22.8	4.25	1,58	<0.05
1 month	29	20.1	18.2	29	38.5	28.8	18.4	5.8 to 31.0	8.47	1,56	<0.01
3 months	29	17.0	17.0	28	28.2	24.8	11.2	0.0 to 22.4	4.00	1,55	<0.05
6 months	29	17.2	14.2	28	29.5	22.1	12.3	2.5 to 22.1	6.25	1,55	<0.05

Table 18 Patient visual analogue scale mean anxiety scores: the future

Time	Treatment			Control			Difference between means	95% confidence interval	F	d.f.	p
	n	Mean	S.D.	n	Mean	S.D.					
24 hours	30	59.2	30.9	30	59.4	27.5	0.2	−14.9 to 15.3	0.00	1,58	n.s.
48 hours	30	45.1	27.8	30	54.8	26.9	9.7	−4.4 to 23.8	1.92	1,58	n.s.
72 hours	30	37.9	24.7	30	52.2	28.2	14.3	0.6 to 28.0	4.40	1,58	<0.05
5 days	30	34.1	24.5	30	52.2	30.6	18.1	3.8 to 32.4	6.37	1,58	<0.01
1 month	29	31.0	26.0	29	50.8	32.0	19.8	4.5 to 35.1	6.73	1,56	<0.01
3 months	29	35.6	25.8	28	43.1	28.8	7.5	−7.0 to 22.0	1.06	1,55	n.s.
6 months	29	32.3	26.6	28	39.1	26.8	6.8	−7.4 to 21.0	0.94	1,55	n.s.

there was a significant reduction for the treatment group compared to controls at 5 days and 1, 3 and 6 months post-infarction.

Spouse anxiety: the future.   Table 20 shows the mean anxiety scores for both groups of spouses on the seven occasions. A one-tailed test revealed that the difference between the groups at baseline (24 hours) was not statistically significant. However, there was a significant reduction for the treatment group compared to controls at 5 days and 1, 3 and 6 months.

Spouse anxiety: sexual activity.   Table 21 shows the mean anxiety scores for both groups of spouses on the seven occasions. A one-tailed test revealed that the difference between the groups at baseline (24 hours) was not statistically significant. However, there was a significant reduction in anxiety in the treatment group compared to controls at 72 hours, 5 days and 1, 3 and 6 months.

Spouse anxiety: general health.   Table 22 shows the mean anxiety scores for both groups of spouses on the seven occasions. A one-tailed test revealed that the difference between the groups at baseline (24 hours) was not statistically significant. However, there was a significant reduction for the treatment group compared to controls at 5 days and 1, 3 and 6 months.

Spouse anxiety: relations with patient.   Table 23 shows the mean anxiety scores for both groups of spouses on the seven occasions. A one-tailed test revealed that the difference between the groups at baseline (24 hours) was not statistically significant. However, there was a significant reduction in anxiety in the treatment group compared to controls at 72 hours, 5 days and 6 months.

Spouse anxiety: ability of patient to work.   Table 24 shows the mean anxiety scores for both groups of spouses on the seven occasions. A one-tailed test revealed that the difference between the groups at baseline (24 hours) was not statistically significant. However, there was a significant reduction for the treatment group compared to controls at 72 hours, 5 days and 1, 3 and 6 months.

Spouse anxiety: another heart attack for patient.   Table 25 shows the mean anxiety scores for both groups of spouses on the seven occasions. A one-tailed test revealed that the difference between the groups at baseline (24 hours) was not statistically significant. However, there was a significant reduction in anxiety in the treatment group compared to controls at 5 days and 1, 3 and 6 months.

Spouse anxiety: possible complications for patient. Table 26 shows the mean anxiety scores for both groups of spouses on the seven occasions. A one-tailed test revealed that the difference between the groups at baseline (24 hours) was not statistically significant. However, there was a significant reduction for the treatment groups compared to controls at 48 hours and 72 hours, 5 days and 1 and 3 months, but not at 6 months.

SATISFACTION

Tables 27 to 30 show the mean satisfaction scores for both groups of patients, while tables 31 to 32 show the scores for both groups of spouses.

Respondents were asked to indicate how satisfied they were with the following factors. Scores ranged from 1 ('not at all satisfied') to 100 ('extremely satisfied').

Patient satisfaction
General health
Table 27 shows the mean satisfaction scores for both groups of patients on the five occasions. A one-tailed test revealed that the difference between the groups at baseline (48 hours) was not statistically significant. However, the treatment group scores remained significantly higher compared to controls at 5 days, 1 month and 6 months post-infarction.

Life in general
Table 28 shows the mean satisfaction scores for both groups of patients on the five occasions. A one-tailed test revealed that the difference between the groups on all occasions was not statistically significant.

Care received
Table 29 shows the mean satisfaction scores for both groups of patients on the five occasions. A one-tailed test revealed that the difference between the groups at baseline (48 hours) was not statistically significant. However, the treatment group scores

Table 19 Spouse visual analogue scale mean anxiety scores: leisure activity

Time	Treatment			Control			Difference between means	95% confidence interval	F	d.f.	p
	n	Mean	S.D.	n	Mean	S.D.					
24 hours	30	46.4	32.9	30	45.7	32.3	−0.7	−17.5 to 16.1	0.01	1,58	n.s.
48 hours	30	33.6	32.8	30	42.2	31.2	8.6	−7.9 to 25.1	1.07	1,58	n.s.
72 hours	30	29.1	29.5	30	41.4	31.3	12.3	−3.4 to 28.0	2.47	1,58	n.s.
5 days	30	25.2	26.1	30	44.7	31.0	19.5	4.7 to 34.3	6.95	1,58	<0.01
1 month	29	22.3	20.6	29	37.6	28.2	15.3	2.3 to 28.3	5.55	1,56	<0.05
3 months	29	18.8	16.6	28	34.6	31.1	15.8	2.6 to 29.0	5.78	1,55	<0.01
6 months	29	18.9	16.1	28	37.6	28.8	18.7	6.4 to 31.0	9.33	1,55	<0.01

Table 20 Spouse visual analogue scale mean anxiety scores: the future

Time	Treatment			Control			Difference between means	95% confidence interval	F	d.f.	p
	n	Mean	S.D.	n	Mean	S.D.					
24 hours	30	52.8	30.7	30	54.4	32.7	1.6	−14.8 to 18.0	0.04	1,58	n.s.
48 hours	30	46.1	28.1	30	50.1	33.4	4.0	−11.9 to 19.9	0.25	1,58	n.s.
72 hours	30	41.7	28.0	30	52.4	32.9	10.7	−5.1 to 26.5	1.84	1,58	n.s.
5 days	30	36.5	23.6	30	52.9	32.8	16.4	1.7 to 31.1	4.94	1,58	<0.05
1 month	29	31.4	25.9	29	47.8	33.4	16.4	0.7 to 32.1	4.32	1,56	<0.05
3 months	29	29.3	26.1	28	47.2	33.5	17.9	2.0 to 33.8	5.06	1,55	<0.05
6 months	29	23.4	22.0	28	42.9	32.4	19.5	4.8 to 34.2	7.09	1,55	<0.01

Table 21 Spouse visual analogue scale mean anxiety scores: sexual activity

Time	Treatment			Control			Difference between means	95% confidence interval	F	d.f.	p
	n	Mean	S.D.	n	Mean	S.D.					
24 hours	30	26.8	25.2	30	26.2	25.7	−0.6	−13.8 to 12.6	0.01	1,58	n.s.
48 hours	30	21.0	24.2	30	27.5	26.9	6.5	−6.7 to 19.7	0.98	1,58	n.s.
72 hours	30	16.5	17.5	30	26.9	27.9	10.4	−1.6 to 22.4	3.01	1,58	<0.05
5 days	30	12.9	15.2	30	29.4	26.4	16.5	4.6 to 28.4	8.77	1,58	<0.01
1 month	29	13.6	17.4	29	24.8	22.7	11.2	0.6 to 21.8	4.47	1,56	<0.05
3 months	29	9.5	7.9	28	26.6	26.2	17.1	6.9 to 27.3	11.33	1,55	<0.001
6 months	29	9.2	8.5	28	22.3	22.2	13.1	4.3 to 21.9	8.77	1,55	<0.01

Table 22 Spouse visual analogue scale mean anxiety scores: general health

Time	Treatment			Control			Difference between means	95% confidence interval	F	d.f.	p
	n	Mean	S.D.	n	Mean	S.D.					
24 hours	30	40.4	30.3	30	39.3	29.9	−1.1	−16.7 to 14.5	0.02	1,58	n.s.
48 hours	30	37.0	30.6	30	34.5	28.6	−2.5	−17.8 to 12.8	0.11	1,58	n.s.
72 hours	30	32.0	26.4	30	37.2	31.7	5.2	−9.9 to 20.3	0.48	1,58	n.s.
5 days	30	28.0	24.9	30	41.5	32.5	13.5	−1.4 to 28.4	3.28	1,58	<0.05
1 month	29	28.1	22.2	29	39.9	30.3	11.8	−2.2 to 25.8	2.84	1,56	<0.05
3 months	29	20.4	16.4	28	37.9	30.3	17.5	4.7 to 30.3	7.38	1,55	<0.01
6 months	29	21.5	20.4	28	34.7	30.8	13.2	−0.6 to 27.0	3.63	1,55	<0.05

Table 23 Spouse visual analogue scale mean anxiety scores: relations with patient

Time	Treatment			Control			Difference between means	95% confidence interval	F	d.f.	p
	n	Mean	S.D.	n	Mean	S.D.					
24 hours	30	26.4	28.2	30	26.8	27.1	0.4	-13.9 to 14.7	0.00	1,58	n.s.
48 hours	30	21.3	25.1	30	27.1	30.4	5.8	-8.6 to 20.2	0.65	1,58	n.s.
72 hours	30	16.2	14.1	30	27.6	29.0	11.4	-0.4 to 23.2	3.77	1,58	<0.05
5 days	30	14.8	14.5	30	29.2	31.1	14.4	1.9 to 26.9	5.30	1,58	<0.05
1 month	29	15.9	21.6	29	22.6	25.5	6.7	-5.7 to 19.1	1.15	1,56	n.s.
3 months	28	15.1	18.0	28	20.9	23.8	5.8	-5.4 to 17.0	1.11	1,55	n.s.
6 months	28	12.4	17.0	28	25.7	26.9	13.3	1.4 to 25.2	5.07	1,55	<0.05

Table 24 Spouse visual analogue scale mean anxiety scores: ability of patient to work

Time	Treatment			Control			Difference between means	95% confidence interval	F	d.f	p
	n	Mean	S.D.	n	Mean	S.D.					
24 hours	30	44.3	35.7	30	42.4	32.8	-1.9	-19.6 to 15.8	0.05	1,58	n.s.
48 hours	30	36.6	31.1	30	43.3	31.9	6.7	-9.5 to 22.2	0.69	1,58	n.s.
72 hours	30	34.7	27.3	30	48.9	29.0	14.2	-0.3 to 28.7	3.83	1,58	<0.05
5 days	30	32.5	28.2	30	49.6	30.7	17.1	1.9 to 32.3	5.06	1,58	<0.05
1 month	29	29.0	21.1	29	51.7	29.8	22.7	9.1 to 36.3	11.14	1,56	<0.001
3 months	29	27.3	17.8	28	52.7	33.8	25.4	11.2 to 39.6	12.76	1,55	<0.001
6 months	29	24.8	20.1	28	41.1	30.2	16.3	2.8 to 29.8	5.79	1,55	<0.01

Table 25 Spouse visual analogue scale mean anxiety scores: another heart attack for patient

Time	Treatment			Control			Difference between means	95% confidence interval	F	d.f.	p
	n	Mean	S.D.	n	Mean	S.D.					
24 hours	30	81.5	23.2	30	79.8	24.6	-1.7	-14.1 to 10.7	0.08	1,58	n.s.
48 hours	30	69.9	28.3	30	77.3	25.3	7.4	-6.4 to 21.2	1.16	1,58	n.s.
72 hours	30	66.5	24.0	30	75.8	25.0	9.3	-3.3 to 21.9	2.13	1,58	n.s.
5 days	30	58.5	24.8	30	76.3	25.1	17.8	4.9 to 37.0	7.59	1,58	<0.01
1 month	29	55.0	25.9	29	70.0	27.3	15.0	1.0 to 29.0	4.57	1,56	<0.05
3 months	29	46.8	26.5	28	61.7	30.5	14.9	-0.2 to 30.0	3.90	1,55	<0.05
6 months	29	43.3	25.2	28	62.9	31.2	19.6	4.6 to 34.6	6.81	1,55	<0.01

Table 26 Spouse visual analogue scale mean anxiety scores: possible complications for patient

Time	Treatment			Control			Difference between means	95% confidence interval	F	d.f	p
	n	Mean	S.D.	n	Mean	S.D.					
24 hours	30	78.4	18.0	30	74.5	19.0	-3.9	-13.4 to 5.6	0.67	1,58	n.s.
48 hours	30	62.2	24.3	30	73.1	19.1	10.9	-0.4 to 22.2	3.77	1,58	<0.05
72 hours	30	62.4	24.3	30	73.1	19.7	10.7	-0.7 to 22.1	3.53	1,58	<0.05
5 days	30	51.6	24.7	30	69.3	27.1	17.7	4.3 to 31.1	7.02	1,58	<0.01
1 month	29	49.4	21.7	29	61.1	30.0	11.7	-2.1 to 25.5	2.89	1,56	<0.05
3 months	29	43.2	24.6	28	59.3	31.8	16.1	1.1 to 31.1	4.62	1,55	<0.05
6 months	29	45.6	25.8	28	56.4	31.2	10.8	-4.4 to 26.0	2.04	1,55	n.s.

Table 27   Patient visual analogue scale mean satisfaction scores: general health

Time	Treatment			Control			Difference between means	95% confidence interval	F	d.f.	p
	n	Mean	S.D.	n	Mean	S.D.					
48 hours	30	66.1	25.6	30	62.5	28.3	3.6	−10.3 to 17.5	0.27	1,58	n.s.
5 days	30	71.1	22.9	30	56.3	28.9	14.8	1.3 to 28.3	4.82	1,58	<0.05
1 month	29	70.5	21.7	29	58.2	29.0	12.3	−1.2 to 25.8	3.34	1,56	<0.05
3 months	29	68.2	23.6	28	62.2	25.6	6.0	−7.0 to 19.0	0.85	1,55	n.s.
6 months	29	72.3	21.4	28	59.7	27.8	12.6	−0.5 to 25.7	3.70	1,55	<0.05

Table 28   Patient visual analogue scale mean satisfaction scores: life in general

Time	Treatment			Control			Difference between means	95% confidence interval	F	d.f.	p
	n	Mean	S.D.	n	Mean	S.D.					
48 hours	30	72.2	22.8	30	74.7	23.4	−2.5	−14.4 to 9.4	0.17	1,58	n.s.
5 days	30	71.7	24.3	30	66.5	22.6	5.2	−6.9 to 17.3	0.74	1,58	n.s.
1 month	29	74.2	21.4	29	68.3	26.2	5.9	−6.6 to 18.4	0.88	1,56	n.s.
3 months	29	73.1	20.1	28	70.9	21.2	2.2	−8.7 to 13.1	0.17	1,55	n.s.
6 months	29	75.5	20.3	28	70.1	22.9	5.4	−6.1 to 16.9	0.91	1,55	n.s.

Table 29 Patient visual analogue scale mean satisfaction scores: care received

Time	Treatment			Control			Difference between means	95% confidence interval	F	d.f	p
	n	Mean	S.D.	n	Mean	S.D.					
48 hours	30	94.4	5.5	30	94.0	4.0	0.4	−2.1 to 2.9	0.07	1,58	n.s.
5 days	30	94.3	5.8	30	89.3	11.4	5.0	0.3 to 9.7	4.51	1,58	<0.05
1 month	29	94.6	6.1	29	91.2	7.3	3.4	−0.1 to 6.9	3.75	1,56	<0.05
3 months	29	95.1	5.2	28	89.6	11.2	5.5	0.9 to 10.1	5.87	1,55	<0.01
6 months	29	95.0	5.6	28	88.7	10.9	6.3	1.7 to 10.9	7.64	1,55	<0.01

Table 30 Patient visual analogue scale mean satisfaction scores: information received

Time	Treatment			Control			Difference between means	95% confidence interval	F	d.f	p
	n	Mean	S.D.	n	Mean	S.D.					
48 hours	30	94.9	5.8	30	90.1	7.9	4.8	1.2 to 8.4	7.10	1,58	<0.01
5 days	30	94.7	4.7	30	87.4	10.7	7.3	3.0 to 11.6	11.41	1,58	<0.001
1 month	29	95.1	5.1	29	84.0	16.4	11.1	4.7 to 17.5	12.17	1,56	<0.001
3 months	29	94.8	6.4	28	79.8	22.0	15.0	6.5 to 23.5	12.45	1,55	<0.001
6 months	29	95.1	4.7	28	79.9	16.8	15.2	8.7 to 21.7	22.24	1,55	<0.001

remained significantly higher than the control group scores at 5 days and 1, 3 and 6 months.

Information received
Table 30 shows the mean satisfaction scores for both groups of patients on the five occasions. A one-tailed test revealed that the difference between groups at baseline (48 hours) was statistically significant. Whereas the control group scores gradually fell over the four other occasions, the treatment group scores remained significantly higher.

Spouse satisfaction

Information received
Table 31 shows the mean satisfaction scores for both groups of spouses on the five occasions. A one-tailed test revealed that the difference between groups at baseline (48 hours) was highly statistically significant. The treatment group scores remained significantly higher than the control group on the other four occasions.

Care patient received
Table 32 shows the mean satisfaction scores for both groups of spouses on the five occasions. A one-tailed test revealed that the difference between groups at baseline (48 hours) was statistically significant. The treatment group scores remained significantly higher than the control group on the four other occasions, markedly so at 5 days and 3 and 6 months.

KNOWLEDGE

Tables 33 and 34 show the mean knowledge scale scores for both groups of patients and spouses respectively.

Patient knowledge
Table 33 shows the mean knowledge scores for both groups of patients on the five occasions. A one-tailed test revealed that the difference between groups at baseline (24 hours) was not statistically significant. However, at follow-up the treatment group scores were significantly higher than the control group scores on each occasion: 5 days and 1, 3 and 6 months.

Table 31 Spouse visual analogue scale mean satisfaction scores: information received

Time	Treatment			Control			Difference between means	95% confidence interval	F	d.f.	p
	n	Mean	S.D.	n	Mean	S.D.					
48 hours	30	95.9	3.8	30	85.3	15.6	10.6	4.7 to 16.5	13.19	1,58	<0.001
5 days	30	96.6	2.6	30	83.8	14.9	12.8	7.3 to 18.3	21.32	1,58	<0.001
1 month	29	96.4	2.4	29	81.8	19.0	14.6	7.5 to 21.7	16.90	1,56	<0.001
3 months	29	95.9	2.3	28	82.2	19.3	13.7	6.5 to 20.9	11.30	1,55	<0.001
6 months	29	95.7	2.3	28	81.0	19.7	14.7	7.3 to 22.1	16.00	1,55	<0.001

Table 32 Spouse visual analogue scale mean satisfaction scores: care patient received

Time	Treatment			Control			Difference between means	95% confidence interval	F	d.f.	p
	n	Mean	S.D.	n	Mean	S.D.					
48 hours	30	96.7	1.9	30	92.9	7.1	3.8	1.1 to 6.5	8.05	1,58	<0.01
5 days	30	97.0	2.1	30	92.5	6.0	4.5	2.2 to 6.8	15.05	1,58	<0.001
1 month	29	96.5	1.8	29	91.5	8.8	5.0	1.7 to 8.3	8.70	1,56	<0.01
3 months	29	96.4	1.8	28	91.3	7.2	5.1	2.4 to 7.8	13.75	1,55	<0.001
6 months	29	96.7	2.1	28	91.8	5.9	4.9	2.6 to 7.2	17.75	1,55	<0.001

Table 33 Patient knowledge questionnaire mean scores

Time	Treatment			Control			Difference between means	95% confidence interval	F	d.f.	p
	n	Mean	S.D.	n	Mean	S.D.					
24 hours	30	6.8	1.6	30	7.3	1.6	−0.5	−1.3 to 0.3	1.72	1,58	n.s.
5 days	30	8.6	1.8	30	7.5	1.4	1.1	0.3 to 1.9	7.29	1,58	<0.01
1 month	29	9.0	1.4	29	7.8	1.6	1.2	0.4 to 2.0	9.05	1,56	<0.01
3 months	29	8.8	1.3	28	7.8	1.5	1.0	0.3 to 1.7	6.99	1,55	<0.01
6 months	29	9.0	1.2	28	7.4	1.5	1.6	0.9 to 2.3	18.70	1,55	<0.001

Table 34 Spouse knowledge questionnaire mean scores

Time	Treatment			Control			Difference between means	95% confidence interval	F	d.f.	p
	n	Mean	S.D.	n	Mean	S.D.					
24 hours	30	7.0	1.6	30	6.8	1.9	0.2	−0.7 to 1.1	0.28	1,58	n.s.
5 days	30	8.8	1.6	30	7.0	1.7	1.8	0.9 to 2.7	16.30	1,58	<0.001
1 month	29	9.4	1.3	29	7.8	1.4	1.6	0.9 to 2.3	21.00	1,56	<0.001
3 months	29	9.4	1.2	28	7.8	1.5	1.6	0.9 to 2.3	18.47	1,55	<0.001
6 months	29	9.0	1.5	28	7.1	1.5	1.9	1.1 to 2.7	22.25	1,55	<0.001

Table 35 Patient activity scale mean scores

Time	Treatment			Control			Difference between means	95% confidence interval	F	d.f.	p
	n	Mean	S.D.	n	Mean	S.D.					
1 month	29	19.2	12.9	29	28.7	26.0	−9.5	−20.2 to 1.2	2.74	1,56	n.s.
3 months	29	27.6	18.6	28	32.0	26.7	−4.4	−16.6 to 7.8	0.55	1,55	n.s.
6 months	29	35.9	20.2	28	39.5	31.9	−3.6	−17.4 to 10.2	0.27	1,55	n.s.

Table 36 Patient mean systolic and diastolic blood pressures (mmHg)

Time	Treatment			Control			Difference between means	95% confidence interval	F	d.f.	p
	n	Mean	S.D.	n	Mean	S.D.					
Systolic:											
24 hours	30	137.1	24.1	30	137.3	22.2	0.2	−11.8 to 12.2	0.00	1,58	n.s.
5 days	30	113.3	11.6	30	117.8	18.9	4.5	−3.6 to 12.6	1.23	1,58	n.s.
6 months	29	128.3	14.2	28	138.8	18.1	10.5	1.9 to 19.1	5.95	1,55	<0.01
Diastolic:											
24 hours	30	90.8	19.3	30	89.3	15.4	−1.5	−10.5 to 7.5	0.11	1,58	n.s.
5 days	30	72.9	9.8	30	72.7	8.2	−0.2	−4.9 to 4.5	0.01	1,58	n.s.
6 months	29	80.2	9.9	28	87.0	11.2	6.8	1.2 to 12.4	5.86	1,55	<0.01

Table 37 Patient mean body mass index (kg/m^2)

Time	Treatment			Control			Difference between means	95% confidence interval	F	d.f.	p
	n	Mean	S.D.	n	Mean	S.D.					
24 hours	30	25.7	2.4	30	25.8	2.8	0.1	−1.3 to 1.5	0.01	1,58	n.s.
1 month	29	25.7	2.7	29	25.5	2.6	−0.2	−1.5 to 1.3	0.04	1,56	n.s.
3months	29	25.7	2.6	28	25.0	2.3	−0.7	−2.0 to 0.6	1.22	1,55	n.s.
6 months	29	25.5	2.5	28	25.5	2.3	0.0	−1.3 to 1.3	0.00	1,55	n.s.

Spouse knowledge

Table 34 shows the mean knowledge scores for both groups of spouses on the five occasions. A one-tailed test revealed that the difference between groups at baseline (24 hours) was not statistically significant. However, at follow-up the treatment group scores were significantly higher than the control group scores on each occasion: 5 days and 1, 3 and 6 months.

ACTIVITY

Table 35 shows the mean activity scores for both groups of patients on the three occasions. A one-tailed test revealed that the difference between groups on each occasion was not statistically significant.

HEALTH DATA

Blood pressure

Table 36 shows the mean systolic and diastolic blood pressures (mmHg) for both groups of patients on the three occasions. A one-tailed test revealed that the difference between groups at baseline (24 hours) was not statistically significant. However, at 6 months the mean systolic and diastolic pressures were statistically significantly lower in the treatment group.

Body mass index

Table 37 shows the mean body mass index (kg/m^2) for both groups of patients on the four occasions. A one-tailed test revealed that the difference between the groups was not statistically significant at baseline (24 hours) or at 1, 3 or 6 months post-infarction.

Tobacco consumption

Smoking behaviour of the patient study groups is depicted in table 38. Prior to admission to hospital, half of each group smoked.

Although at the 1-month follow-up only one person in each group claimed still to be smoking, this figure increased at each follow-up period, roughly twice as much in the control group. However, a comparison of the results using a chi-square test revealed that there were no statistically significant differences between the two groups.

Table 38 Smoking characteristics of the study groups

Variable	Treatment	Control	x^2	d.f.	p
Number of patients smoking:					
Prior to admission	15	17	0.26	1	n.s.
At 1 month	1	1	0.00	1	n.s.
At 3 months	2	4	0.25	1	n.s.
At 6 months	5	8	1.02	1	n.s.

EMPLOYMENT STATUS

Employment characteristics of the study groups are shown in table 39. Prior to admission to hospital, three patients (one unemployed and two retired) in the treatment group and four (one unemployed and three retired) in the control group were not in employment. At the completion of the study, eight patients in the treatment group and five in the control group had not returned to work. A comparison of the results using a chi-square test revealed that there were no statistically significant differences between the two groups.

Table 39 Employment characteristics of the study groups

Variable	Treatment	Control	x^2	d.f.	p
Number of patients working:					
Prior to admission	27	26	0.15	1	n.s.
At 3 months	13	13	0.14	1	n.s.
At 6 months	17	16	0.13	1	n.s.
Early retirement	1	3	0.13	1	n.s.

PHYSICAL STATE

Angina

Table 40 shows the number of patients in each study group reporting angina at follow-up. Between discharge from the hospital and the 1-month follow up, it can be seen that, compared to the treatment group, twice as many patients in the control group were experiencing angina on moderate to severe exertion. Angina on mild exertion and at rest was relatively infrequent and similar in both groups. Using ranking techniques as described by Meddis (1980, 1984), a one-tailed test revealed that this difference reached statistical significance.

Table 40 Patients with angina* in the study groups

Variable	Treatment	Control	
At 1 month:			
Nil	20	13	
Grade 1	6	13	
Grade 2	2	1	$z = 1.63, p = 0.05$
Grade 3	1	2	
Total	29	29	
At 3 months:			
Nil	17	14	
Grade 1	10	11	
Grade 2	2	3	$z = 0.70, p > 0.10$
Grade 3	–	–	
Total	29	28	
At 6 months:			
Nil	16	17	
Grade 1	13	7	
Grade 2	–	4	$z = 0.06, p > 0.10$
Grade 3	–	–	
Total	29	28	

*Grades of angina: 1 = On moderate/severe exertion
2 = On mild exertion
3 = At rest

At the 3- and 6-month follow-ups, the difference between groups on grades of angina was not statistically significant.

It can be seen from table 40 that between one third and one half of all the patients in each group were still experiencing some degree of angina 6 months after discharge from the hospital.

Dyspnoea

Table 41 shows the number of patients in each study group reporting dyspnoea at follow-up. Roughly one half of all patients in each group were experiencing some degree of dyspnoea, predominantly on moderate to severe exertion, between discharge from the hospital and the 6-month follow-up appointment.

Table 41   Patients with dyspnoea* in the study groups

Variables	Treatment	Control	
At 1 month:			
Nil	17	16	
Grade 1	9	10	
Grade 2	3	2	$z = 0.25, p > 0.10$
Grade 3	–	1	
Total	29	29	
At 3 months:			
Nil	12	15	
Grade 1	15	11	
Grade 2	2	1	$z = -0.79, p > 0.10$
Grade 3	–	1	
Total	29	28	
At 6 months:			
Nil	14	16	
Grade 1	12	8	
Grade 2	2	3	$z = -0.43, p > 0.10$
Grade 3	1	1	
Total	29	28	

*Grades of dyspnoea: 1 = On moderate/severe exertion
                       2 = On mild exertion
                       3 = At rest

Although the number of patients in each group reporting dyspnoea was similar at 1 month post-infarction, it became higher in the treatment group at 3 and 6 months. However, a one-tailed test revealed that these differences were not statistically significant.

Morbidity

Table 42 depicts data on patient in-hospital morbidity, reinfarction and readmission rates for both study groups.

Table 42 Patient morbidity in the study groups

Variable	Treatment	Control
In-hospital morbidity:		
Cardiac arrest	1	1
Complete heart block	1	–
Reinfarction:		
Between discharge and 1 month follow-up	1	–
Between 1-month and 6-month follow-ups	–	–
Readmission:		
Between discharge and 1-month follow-up	2	2
Between 1-month and 3-month follow-ups	1	1
Between 3-month and 6-month follow-ups	1	–

The major in-hospital cardiovascular morbidity was from cardiac arrest occurring in two patients while in the CCU. The other major event was the occurrence of complete heart block in one of the treatment group while in the CCU. This patient required the insertion of a temporary pacing wire, which was *in situ* for less than 48 hours.

Only one patient had a reinfarction, which occurred 3 weeks after discharge and was diagnosed following readmission to a medical ward when the patient had complained of vague chest discomfort.

Altogether, seven patients required readmission to hospital. Apart from the patient described above, the reasons for readmission included investigations and/or management of heart failure (n = 3), pulmonary embolism (n = 1), deep vein thrombosis (n = 1) and non-cardiac problems (n = 2).

Statistical analysis was thought to be inappropriate here because of the similarities between groups and the small numbers involved.

7 Discussion

The results from this study provide evidence to support the overall contention that a programme of in-hospital nursing support can confer additional benefits over and above the management regimen for coronary patients and their spouses. The findings from this study support all three of the original hypotheses (p.27). The study demonstrates that a simple programme of in-hospital counselling, provided by a coronary care registered nurse, statistically significantly reduces anxiety and depression, and increases satisfaction and knowledge, in male coronary patients and their spouses.

This study has provided a systematic assessment of educative-supportive counselling in a well-defined group. An important consideration in the design was the selection of a homogeneous sample with respect to sex, cardiological status and location of care.

QUALITY OF STUDY DESIGN

In order to check the level of quality of this research design, the author compared it with the Methodology Quality Rating system devised by Padgett et al (1988), based upon the work of Sackett and Haynes (1976). According to this system, rating points (up to a maximum of 16) are awarded to a study depending on how well it addresses basic issues of internal and external validity. Padgett and her colleagues used this rating system in a meta-analysis of the effects of educational and psychosocial interventions on management of diabetes mellitus. They found that the rated quality of research design in 93 studies ranged from 2 to 14 points, with an average score of 7.5 points.

Using the Methodology Quality Rating system, this study met the following requirements:

1.   Design of study/assignment (internal validity)
The study obtained the maximum score of 5 points in this section, as it satisfied the following criteria:

- Experimental design with random assignment (3 points).
- Treatment and control groups are specified as equivalent on three or more variables (1 point).
- Attrition rate less than 15% (1 point).

2.   Selection and specification of study sample (external validity)
The study obtained 5 out of a possible 6 points in this section, as it satisfied the following criteria:

- Systematic sample from specified population (1 point).
- Clearly replicable diagnostic criteria (1 point).
- Dropouts described (1 point).
- Three or more sample characteristics described (1 point).
- Inclusion/exclusion criteria specified (1 point). It was not a random sample of all subjects from a specified population.

3.   Other methodological features
The study obtained the maximum of 5 points in this section, as it satisfied the following criteria:

- Potential confounding variables are specified and measured (any number) (1 point).
- Blinding specified and used (1 point).
- Ratings of outcomes (75 to 100%) (3 points).

Thus, using this method of quality rating, the present study achieves a score of 15 out of a possible total of 16. This score compares very favourably with the average score of 7.5 and the highest score of 14 awarded by Padgett et al to the 93 studies they reviewed.

Although a double-blind trial of counselling would be the ideal research design, its achievement is fraught with practical difficulties. It was an important consideration of this study that the therapist was blind to any data obtained by the other researcher.

DISCUSSION OF SPECIFIC FINDINGS

Anxiety and depression

Mean anxiety scores for the patients and spouses were high at 24 hours and generally decreased over the study period. However, although the scores were similar at baseline, they were generally statistically significantly lower in the treatment group at each stage of follow-up. Mean depression scores for the patients and spouses were generally low in both groups, although the patient treatment group reported less depression than the controls up to 3 months after leaving hospital.

Anxiety and depression are notoriously difficult to measure. Study findings are dependent upon the type and timing of the measurement tools used. Use of the Hospital Anxiety and Depression (HAD) scale seemed to prove highly satisfactory: respondents appeared to find the instrument easy and quick to complete. Unlike most other anxiety or depression scales, the HAD scale has no items relating to somatic symptoms that may be due to physical illness, even in the absence of clinical anxiety or depression. Many previous studies of anxiety and depression in medical patients have used rating measures emphasising somatic symptoms such as insomnia and weight loss, which are common in physical illness even without mood disturbance, and are likely to overestimate the prevalence of anxiety and depression (Schwab et al, 1967). The HAD scale, designed to assess anxiety and depression in physically ill patients and validated in such groups, would be expected to yield more conservative and also more accurate estimates.

The HAD scale mean scores for patient anxiety and depression and spouse anxiety had dramatically decreased from baseline to 5 days in the treatment group, whereas the scores in the control group remained the same or even increased slightly. From 5 days to 6 months there was a gradual decline of scores in both groups at each follow-up phase, which were generally significantly lower in the treatment group. Spouse depression scores decreased more in the treatment group, but the difference was not statistically significant.

The use of visual analogue scales also proved to be highly satisfactory. Again, respondents seemed to have no difficulty in completing these instruments. McCormack et al (1988) provide evidence that visual analogue scales are not only well suited to experimental designs employing repeated measures and within-subject comparisons, but also successfully discriminate in between-subject studies.

The relative magnitudes of the mean scores of each visual analogue scale show that patients and spouses in both study groups were initially particularly anxious about the possibility of another heart attack for the patients and, to a lesser extent, their general health and the future in general. In addition, spouses reported being particularly anxious about the possibility of complications for the patient. These findings are in general agreement with earlier work by the researcher (Thompson et al, 1982, 1987; Thompson and Cordle, 1988). However, respondents may have been anxious about other specific factors that were not covered by these scales.

Prior to discharge from hospital, patients in the treatment group were statistically significantly less anxious about their general health, ability to resume work and leisure activities, the possible occurrence of complications and the future in general than were controls. After discharge home, patients in the treatment group were less anxious about suffering another heart attack, relations with their spouse and resuming leisure activities. Spouses in the treatment group were statistically significantly less anxious than were controls on all of the variables measured, and virtually all of these differences were sustained at each follow-up period. Thus, these findings seem to suggest that the programme of support is particularly beneficial for the spouse. A possible explanation for this is the disparity between the level of counselling provided for the spouses in the two study groups. In other words, the provision of in-hospital routine support for spouses, in contrast to that for their partners, is typically scant, whereas the spouses in the treatment groups received fairly detailed support, similar to that of their partners.

Interestingly, the HAD scale and many of the visual analogue scale mean scores for spouse anxiety were higher on each occasion than were those for patient anxiety. For instance, spouses were more anxious about the possibility of another heart attack and/or complications for the patient, relations and sexual activity with the patient and leisure activity. These findings indicate either that spouses are more anxious than patients or that women are more anxious than men. Vetter et al (1977) found that women admitted to a CCU were more anxious than men, and Cay (1982) reported that wives were more anxious than their husbands, at least during the acute phase of the illness. The reasons for this are unclear. However, the diagnosis, suddenness and perception of a heart attack pose a devastating threat to physical, personal and psychological well-being, creating a crisis for the spouse as well as for the patient (Skelton and Dominian, 1973; Mayou et al, 1978a). In the immediate period after patients are discharged from hospital, many spouses perceive their husbands as vulnerable and are often uncertain of what they should do to care for them. This may explain why spouse anxiety is high. An alternative explanation is that although counselling was provided to the couple, each partner provided mutual support to the other. The patient may be less anxious because of the support and education received not only from the nurse but also from his well-informed and prepared spouse. However, it is worth noting that all coronary patients, including those in the present study, were routinely prescribed beta-adrenergic receptor blocking agents; in addition to the effect of these drugs on the cardiovascular system, the effect on autonomic arousal may have masked the true level of patient anxiety (Peet, 1988).

Satisfaction

The need to assess consumer satisfaction is assuming increasing prominence in health-care evaluation. Patients' and spouses' satisfaction with various aspects of the care they receive is not only a desirable goal in its own right but is an important determinant of compliance and adherence to advice (Ley, 1988).

Patient satisfaction with the levels of health and life in general was relatively high, stable and similar in both groups, and mean satisfaction scores concerning the levels of care and information received were extremely high. This might be explained by low expectations and general satisfaction with virtually any level of care or by the fact that the subjects were aware that they were included in a study. However, despite the brevity and simplicity of the treatment package, it enhanced couple satisfaction, as the scores in the treatment group were consistently and statistically significantly higher, with considerably less scatter, as reflected by the small standard deviations.

The directions of change of the satisfaction scores over the seven occasions in both groups are interesting. There was a general decrease for the patients and spouses of the control group regarding satisfaction with the care and information received, whereas in the treatment group, the scores were either maintained or increased, even at 6 months after leaving hospital. Perhaps the counselling made the couples more confident, less anxious and thus more satisfied. Interestingly, there appears to be close agreement between the patients and spouses concerning satisfaction with information and care received. Thus, it appears that couples have a lasting impression of how satisfied they were with the care and information provided to them.

Knowledge

Patients' and spouses' knowledge scores increased during the patients' stay in the hospital and were retained, and indeed higher, after discharge home. Although both control and treatment groups acquired information about their condition and management, the treatment group, especially the spouses, was the more knowledgeable.

The knowledge questionnaire was a simple instrument that measured only a limited number of subject areas. It is possible that after completion of the first questionnaire, respondents became aware of certain deficits in knowledge and those in the treatment group had the opportunity to target discussion around these areas at subsequent counselling sessions.

Of course, there was no control of patients or spouses actively seeking information after discharge. Even if this accounted for the findings at 1 and 3 months post-infarction, it is unlikely to account for those at 6 months, when the couple completed the instruments in the CCU in the presence of the researchers.

Activity

The activity scores of both groups of patients increased at each follow-up stage. The treatment group consistently reported lower levels of general physical activity than did the control group. However, the difference was not statistically significant, and over the three intervals, the gap in mean scores between the groups narrowed. The rating scale used was a rather crude instrument, and it might have been useful to examine physical, leisure and sexual activity, rather than making a global assessment.

It is debatable whether or not the measurement of activity levels was an appropriate yardstick for assessing recovery because the intervention programme emphasised the importance of adequate rest and the gradual resumption of activity. Thus, early return to pre-infarction levels of activity might not necessarily be indicative of successful outcome.

Physical measures

Smoking
Half of patients in each study group smoked prior to admission to the hospital. Cessation of smoking initially appeared dramatic in that only one patient in either group claimed to be smoking after 1 month. However, this figure doubled at 3 and 6 months, roughly twice as much in the control group. Thus, two-thirds of smokers in the treatment group stopped, compared to just over half of the control group. Accuracy of patient reports was difficult to assess, and reliance was placed on spouse reporting to ensure some reliability. Although data on smoking were obtained by self-report, reliability was considerably enhanced at the 6-month follow-up by the use of expired air carbon monoxide sampling.

It would have been interesting to have obtained data on the smoking characteristics of spouses. Couples in the treatment group received counselling on cessation of smoking, and possibly spouses would have been motivated to give up, as well as being able to provide encouragement to their partners.

Blood pressure
One would expect a fall in blood pressure over the duration of hospital stay due to bedrest and generally reduced activity. Following discharge, a rise to near pre-admission levels would also be normally expected. However, the significant reduction in both systolic and diastolic blood pressure in the treatment group at the 6-month follow-up is a surprising finding. Indirect systolic and diastolic blood pressure measurements were recorded by the same nurse, using an electronic monitor with digital readout, thereby

reducing the possibility of observer error. Thus, it seems reasonable to suggest that the programme exerts an important influence on the cardiovascular system. A possible explanation for this effect could be that patients were given general advice about the importance of 'slowing down' and taking rest periods after meals.

Body mass index
It was, perhaps, not surprising that the body mass index was similar in both groups. The mean group scores remained relatively stable. They were consistently within the upper limits of the normal range and therefore necessitated little intervention in terms of weight reduction.

Return to work

After 3 months, half of the patients in each study group had returned to work. By 6 months nearly 60% of each group were back at work. Rates of return to work vary. For example, Mayberry et al (1983) and Trelawny-Ross and Russell (1986) found that at 6 months about half of the male coronary patients who had been employed full time before being admitted to hospital were back at work. Other researchers, such as Naismith et al (1979) and Maeland and Havik (1987), have found much higher percentages of their samples (88% and 73% respectively) returning to work 6 months post-infarction.

Factors such as angina and breathlessness may account for the findings, although, at 6 months, the remaining patients in both groups stated that they were actively seeking full employment, even though this was proving difficult because of the bleak employment climate.

Morbidity

The number of patients reporting angina was statistically significantly lower in the treatment group at the 1-month follow-up, although by 3 and 6 months the differences were not significant, with between one third and one half of all patients reporting angina. Similar numbers of patients were reporting dyspnoea. However, these rates are less than those of other studies, such as Winefield and Martin (1981) who found that 65% of their sample were reporting such symptoms.

Reinfarction and mortality

The programme did not affect death or reinfarction rates. However, the mortality (5%) and reinfarction (1.6%) rates were extremely low in this study, possibly because the patients selected were classed as mildly or moderately ill. Because of these low figures, it was unlikely that a statistically significant difference would be revealed.

The attrition rate in this study was exceptionally low (5%) and wholly explained by deaths.

GENERAL DISCUSSION

This study is one of very few that provide a detailed and systematic evaluation of a programme of support for coronary patients and spouses. Moreover, it is the only study to date that has specifically evaluated the programme during the patients' stay in hospital.

Although various acute-phase studies of coronary patients report generally positive outcomes, there are serious methodological and/or reporting problems (Razin, 1985). For instance, most studies lack controls or are purely anecdotal. Others inadequately describe their methods, assessments and analyses. Many have used only one or two outcome criteria, such as return to work, mortality or level of anxiety or depression. Although all of these are undoubtedly relevant, a combination of various criteria is needed to gain a more accurate and complete picture.

The findings of this study are in agreement with those reviewed by Mumford et al (1982), providing strong evidence attesting to the efficacy of psychological intervention for individuals faced with stressful, or even physically traumatic, events. In their meta-analytical review, Mumford et al classified the interventions according to whether they offered mainly educational and informational preparation or whether they used psychotherapeutic approaches designed primarily to give emotional support. When averaging the effect sizes, they concluded that the therapeutic approaches appeared more effective but that interventions combining both approaches were superior to either one used singly.

In this study, the treatment package was comprehensive, and thus the differential impact of education and emotional support remains unclear. As Mumford et al (1982) point out in their review, the efficacy of providing both educational and emotional support may simply reflect increased chances of meeting the needs of more couples when two different types of intervention are offered.

The findings of this controlled trial compare favourably with those of previous in-hospital studies (Gruen, 1975; Langosch et al, 1982; Oldenburg et al, 1985). This study lends further support to the conclusions of Perkins et al (1986) that there is now accumulating evidence to demonstrate that in-hospital psychological and educational interventions with first myocardial infarction patients in the days immediately following the infarction favourably influence psychological outcome. Indeed, it is possible that, as Oldenburg et al (1985) suggested in their discussion, the effects of the intervention might have been underestimated, as there were a number of factors that mitigated against significant findings. Other than the major selection criteria of patients having to be younger than 66 years of age, living with a partner and having had a documented first, uncomplicated myocardial infarction, patients were included irrespective of their likely suitability for psychological and/or educational intervention. On balance, the study population can be considered as fairly representative of those patients admitted to a coronary care unit with an uncomplicated heart attack.

A novel feature of this study was the inclusion of the spouse at this early stage of management and the effect of the intervention on the spouse's reported anxiety level. The important role of the spouse in the patient's adjustment during convalescence and her influence on the rate and extent of the patient's recovery is well recognised (Mayou et al, 1978a, b, c). Mayou et al concluded that more practical help and advice should be provided for wives of coronary patients during the hospital phase. Stern and Pascale (1979) specifically suggested that an in-hospital education or psychological therapy group for couples might prove beneficial. Despite such recommendations, no systematic study of the effects of such interventions on anxiety, depression, satisfaction and knowledge have been reported until now. Spouses have been virtually ignored in acute-phase intervention studies, despite the fact that successful patient recovery hinges largely on their education and involvement.

The present study demonstrates that the impact of the myocardial infarction and the programme of support was as great on the spouse. In fact, the inclusion of the spouse in such programmes seems vital in view of the higher levels of reported anxiety.

The effects of the intervention programme on patient anxiety and depression and partner depression are quite dramatic considering they occurred over a period of roughly 4 days from the start of the intervention. Indeed, they occurred after only three half-hour sessions of counselling, as the follow-up measurements were obtained prior to the fourth session of counselling, which took place at 5 days. Although spouse depression decreased over the 4 days in the intervention groups, and increased in the control group, the differences were not statistically significant.

IMPLICATIONS FOR PRACTICE

Conclusions on the relative efficacy of treatment are typically based on statistical evaluation of outcomes. However, in clinical trials, where alternative treatments are compared, the primary interest is in clinical outcome. It is of value to show that there is some clear benefit of a more practical nature favouring one treatment over another.

If the findings in the present study are shown on replication to be robust, they are likely to have important implications for the ways in which in-hospital recovery programmes should be devised for coronary care units.

As Wilson-Barnett (1984) has pointed out,

'progress in the research field is sadly not reflected in levels of clinical implementation of these interventions by nurses' (p.70).

Nichols (1984) has eloquently described some of the objections and criticisms offered by nurses for why they cannot provide this sort of support on a routine basis, for example 'Nurses are too busy' and 'We just do not have the time or staff'. Nichols (1985) labels these 'the problems of psychological neglect' (p.231).

Against the background, a preliminary summary of the research findings was presented to all the staff of the CCU where the study was carried out. This presentation was well received, and the programme of couple counselling certainly appears to have been incorporated into routine clinical practice.

The package of care described in this study is simple, easy to implement and takes up little time − about 2 hours over a 1-week period for each couple. It also requires little investment in training personnel and none in additional staff, finances or other resources, but means that nursing time can be spent more effectively and efficiently for patient and spouse welfare.

Implementing this type of intervention is likely to increase nurses' job satisfaction because they are actually doing something that has been scientifically shown to be beneficial. The necessary patient and spouse involvement, with increased responsibility, might further enhance professional worth. Developing such a role on a routine basis is likely to clarify the nurse's own position in an environment that has become technically and medically orientated.

It is suggested that appropriate, well-timed psychological intervention in the acute phase is therapeutically beneficial, efficient and economic. It is useful on humanitarian as well as medical grounds, giving patients a share in the responsibility for their own care rather than a complete dependence on health professionals. Therefore, it should be routinely offered to first-time coronary patients and their partners.

LIMITATIONS OF THE RESEARCH

An obvious limitation of this study is that the findings are only directly applicable to male patients aged less than 66 years who have suffered a first uncomplicated heart attack.

Once discharged from hospital, the patient and spouse are likely to receive or seek additional information and support from other sources, including friends, literature and the media. Obviously, this would prove exceedingly difficult to control for, or indeed measure, and one has to assume that both the control and treatment groups would have undertaken such activity on an equal basis.

The 1-, 3-, and 6-month follow-up times were selected on a fairly arbitrary basis. However, because mean anxiety and depression scores decreased quite significantly for both the treatment and control groups from their hospital stay to the 1-month follow-up, with only a slight further decline at the 3- and 6-month periods, it appears that major psychosocial adjustments are generally dealt with by the patient during the first month post-infarction. Certainly, following an uncomplicated first heart attack, the patient should be able to resume involvement in work, social and domestic activity within 3 months of leaving hospital. In any case, there are drawbacks, such as reduced compliance, to collecting detailed data at frequent intervals.

Clearly, the individual who wishes to implement such a programme of counselling must have the necessary knowledge and skills, and a genuine desire to initiate the programme, in an attempt to gain credibility in order positively to influence the couple, otherwise the efficacy of the programme will be in doubt. The quality of the relationship with the couple is likely to be an important factor in successful counselling. This has to involve trust, respect, understanding and interest. Coronary care nurses, by virtue of such involvement on a frequent basis, are ideally suited to undertake such a role.

RECOMMENDATIONS FOR FURTHER RESEARCH

It is suggested that the study be replicated in other coronary care units and medical wards. Follow up to at least beyond 6-months and preferably 1 year would provide information on whether or not the effects are sustained over the long term.

An interesting study would be to provide the spouse alone with the counselling programme to examine whether or not this has any significant impact on the patient as well as the spouse.

Another design feature that might be incorporated is to extend the treatment to the couple during the first few months of convalescence, to see if continued support on a routine basis might reduce reported angina, dyspnoea and emotional distress and therefore facilitate an earlier and/or improved return to previous life.

It would be interesting to replicate the study with female coronary patients and their male partners and examine whether the degree of emotional distress is different.

It would also be useful to identify and evaluate the principal active ingredients of the package. Elimination of those components that make no contribution might ensure that a more compact and efficacious intervention is achieved.

Research has not yet made clear the particular aspects of psychological intervention that are responsible for the improved physical or psychosocial functioning.

SUMMARY

This study was designed to assess the efficacy of an in-hospital programme of supportive-educative counselling for male first-time coronary patients and their spouses. It has shown that such a programme, provided by a coronary care registered nurse, can favourably affect psychological well-being in both partners during the hospital stay and after discharge home.

The package of support described appears therapeutic and economical. It seems reasonable to suggest that at least all male first coronary patients and their spouses should be offered a treatment package that comprises supportive-educative counselling.

Appendix I
Intervention guidelines

Prior to *each* intervention, ascertain the couple's level of understanding and whether they have any problems they wish to discuss. Reinforce information, clarify issues and correct misconceptions.

1. 24 HOURS (CCU)

- Reason for admission:
    Patient understanding of problem(s)
    Information about heart attack
    Symptoms to be reported
- Purpose of CCU:
    Rationale for observation and management
    Likely outcome
    Length of stay
    Staff
    Equipment
    General environment
- Daily routines:
    Plan and pattern of day
    Ward rounds
    Visiting hours
- Observations:
    Cardiac monitoring
    Blood pressure
    Temperature
    Respirations
- Medications and intravenous infusions:
    Insertion of intravenous cannulae
    Narcotic analgesic agents

      Antiemetic agents
      Antiarrhythmic agents
      Nitrate therapy, including GTN
- Oxygen:
      Nasal cannulae for administration
      No smoking
- Activity:
      Leg exercises
      Breathing exercises
      Bedrest – commode and urinal, washbowl
      Graduated mobility – toilet and shower
- Investigations:
      Chest X-ray
      ECG
      Blood samples
- Diet:
      Small, frequent meals
      High fibre
      Avoid food high in saturated fat or salt
- Personal problems:
      Job and financial worries
      Concern about family
- Emotional reactions:
      Fear, apprehension and anxiety
- Possible referral to other health/social agencies:
      Social worker
      Dietitian
      Clinical psychologist
- Brief summary
- Opportunity for questions

2. 48 HOURS (CCU)

- Basic structure and function of the heart:
      Coronary blood supply
- Development of ischaemic heart disease:
      Atherosclerosis
      Plaque formation
- Acute myocardial infarction:
      Risk factors

        Warning signs and symptoms
        Healing process
        Personal response
- Activity planning:
        Graduated mobility
- Preparation for transfer to ward:
        Sign of progress
        New environment and routines
        Different nursing and medical staff
        Change in staff:patient ratio
        Discontinue cardiac monitoring
- Possible mood changes:
        Anxiety and depression
        Feelings of guilt and loneliness in spouse
        Avoidance of overprotectiveness by spouse
- Brief summary
- Opportunity for questions

3. 72 HOURS (WARD)

- Family, occupational, social and financial concerns:
        Sickness benefit
        Old age pension
        PSV/HGV licence holders to inform DVLC
- Pertinent life-style and possible modifications:
        Dietary recommendations
        Weight reduction
        Smoking cessation
        Regular health examination
        Adequate rest periods and 'slowing down'
        Avoidance of engagement in multiple activities
- Medications:
        Level of understanding
        Need for compliance
- Activity planning:
        Work
        Leisure
        Sexual
- Brief summary
- Opportunity for questions

4.   5 DAYS (WARD)

- Possible adjustments to be made regarding homecoming
- Activity planning (reinforcement)
- Pertinent life-style modifications (reinforcement)
- Medications (reinforcement)
- Anticipate potential problems:
    Angina
    Shortness of breath
    Lethargy/fatigue
    Sleeplessness
    Poor concentration
    Mood changes
    Somatic problems in spouse
    Strain on marital relations
- Summoning appropriate help:
    Who, when, and how
- CCU telephone number for contact
- Out-patient clinic appointments
- Possible referral to other expert agencies:
    General practitioner
    District nurse
- Brief summary
- Opportunity for questions

Appendix II
Eysenck Personality Questionnaire (EPQ)

Occupation...

Age......................... Sex....................

INSTRUCTIONS Please answer each question by putting a circle around the '**YES**' or the '**NO**' following the question. There are no right or wrong answers, and no trick questions. Work quickly and do not think too long about the exact meaning of the questions.

PLEASE REMEMBER TO ANSWER EACH QUESTION

1	Do you have many different hobbies?	YES	NO
2	Do you stop to think things over before doing anything?	YES	NO
3	Does your mood often go up and down?	YES	NO
4	Have you ever taken the praise for something you knew someone else had really done?........	YES	NO
5	Are you a talkative person?	YES	NO
6	Would being in debt worry you?................	YES	NO
7	Do you ever feel 'just miserable' for no reason? ..	YES	NO
8	Were you ever greedy by helping yourself to more than your share of anything?..............	YES	NO
9	Do you lock up your house carefully at night? ...	YES	NO
10	Are you rather lively?	YES	NO
11	Would it upset you a lot to see a child or an animal suffer?	YES	NO
12	Do you often worry about things you should not have done or said?	YES	NO
13	If you say you will do something, do you always keep your promise no matter how inconvenient it might be?	YES	NO

14 Can you usually let yourself go and enjoy yourself at a lively party? .... YES   NO

15 Are you an irritable person? .... YES   NO

16 Have you ever blamed someone for doing something you knew was really your fault? ...... YES   NO

17 Do you enjoy meeting new people? .... YES   NO

18 Do you believe insurance schemes are a good idea? .... YES   NO

19 Are your feelings easily hurt? .... YES   NO

20 Are *all* your habits good and desirable ones? ..... YES   NO

21 Do you tend to keep in the background on social occasions? .... YES   NO

22 Would you take drugs which may have strange or dangerous effects? .... YES   NO

23 Do you often feel 'fed-up'? .... YES   NO

24 Have you ever taken anything (even a pin or button) that belonged to someone else? .... YES   NO

25 Do you like going out a lot? .... YES   NO

26 Do you enjoy hurting people you love? .... YES   NO

27 Are you often troubled about feelings of guilt? ... YES   NO

28 Do you sometimes talk about things you know nothing about? .... YES   NO

29 Do you prefer reading to meeting people? .... YES   NO

30 Do you have enemies who want to harm you? ... YES   NO

31 Would you call yourself a nervous person? ...... YES   NO

32 Do you have many friends? .... YES   NO

33 Do you enjoy practical jokes that can sometimes really hurt people? .... YES   NO

34 Are you a worrier? .... YES   NO

35 As a child did you do as you were told immediately and without grumbling? .... YES   NO

36 Would you call yourself happy-go-lucky? .... YES   NO

37 Do good manners and cleanliness matter much to you? .... YES   NO

38 Do you worry about awful things that might happen? .... YES   NO

39 Have you ever broken or lost something belonging to someone else? .... YES   NO

40 Do you usually take the initiative in making new friends? .... YES   NO

41 Would you call yourself tense or 'highly-strung'? YES   NO

42 Are you mostly quiet when you are with other people? .... YES NO

43 Do you think marriage is old-fashioned and should be done away with? .... YES NO

44 Do you sometimes boast a little? .... YES NO

45 Can you easily get some life into a rather dull party? .... YES NO

46 Do people who drive carefully annoy you? ...... YES NO

47 Do you worry about your health? .... YES NO

48 Have you ever said anything bad or nasty about anyone? .... YES NO

49 Do you like telling jokes and funny stories to your friends? .... YES NO

50 Do most things taste the same to you? .... YES NO

51 As a child were you ever cheeky to your parents? YES NO

52 Do you like mixing with people? .... YES NO

53 Does it worry you if you know there are mistakes in your work? .... YES NO

54 Do you suffer from sleeplessness? .... YES NO

55 Do you always wash before a meal? .... YES NO

56 Do you nearly always have a 'ready answer' when people talk to you? .... YES NO

57 Do you like to arrive at appointments in plenty of time? .... YES NO

58 Have you often felt listless and tired for no reason? .... YES NO

59 Have you ever cheated at a game? .... YES NO

60 Do you like doing things in which you have to act quickly? .... YES NO

61 Is (or was) your mother a good woman? .... YES NO

62 Do you often feel life is very dull? .... YES NO

63 Have you ever taken advantage of someone? .... YES NO

64 Do you often take on more activities than you have time for? .... YES NO

65 Are there several people who keep trying to avoid you? .... YES NO

66 Do you worry a lot about your looks? .... YES NO

67 Do you think people spend too much time safeguarding their future with savings and insurances? .... YES NO

68 Have you ever wished that you were dead? ...... YES NO

69 Would you dodge paying taxes if you were sure
    you could never be found out? .... YES   NO
70 Can you get a party going? .... YES   NO
71 Do you try not to be rude to people? .... YES   NO
72 Do you worry too long after an embarrassing
    experience? .... YES   NO
73 Have you ever insisted on having your own way? YES   NO
74 When you catch a train do you often arrive at the
    last minute? .... YES   NO
75 Do you suffer from 'nerves'? .... YES   NO
76 Do your friendships break up easily without it
    being your fault? .... YES   NO
77 Do you often feel lonely? .... YES   NO
78 Do you always practise what you preach? .... YES   NO
79 Do you sometimes like teasing animals? .... YES   NO
80 Are you easily hurt when people find fault with
    you or the work you do? .... YES   NO
81 Have you ever been late for an appointment or
    work? .... YES   NO
82 Do you like plenty of bustle and excitement
    around you? .... YES   NO
83 Would you like other people to be afraid of you? . YES   NO
84 Are you sometimes bubbling over with energy
    and sometimes very sluggish? .... YES   NO
85 Do you sometimes put off until tomorrow what
    you ought to do today? .... YES   NO
86 Do other people think of you as being very lively? YES   NO
87 Do people tell you a lot of lies? .... YES   NO
88 Are you touchy about some things? .... YES   NO
89 Are you always willing to admit it when you
    have made a mistake? .... YES   NO
90 Would you feel very sorry for an animal caught in
    a trap? .... YES   NO

**PLEASE CHECK TO SEE THAT YOU HAVE ANSWERED ALL
THE QUESTIONS**

(Reproduced by kind permission of H.J. Eysenck and S.B.G.
Eysenck.)

Appendix III
Hospital Anxiety and
Depression (HAD) scale

Name: Date:

Doctors are aware that emotions play an important part in most illnesses. If your doctor knows about these feelings he will be able to help you more.

This questionnaire is designed to help your doctor to know how you feel. Read each item and place a firm tick in the box opposite the reply which comes closest to how you have been feeling in the past week.

Don't take too long over your replies: your immediate reaction to each item will probably be more accurate than a long thought-out response.

Tick only one box in each section

I feel tense or 'wound up':

Most of the time ....

A lot of the time ....

Time to time, Occasionally.........

Not at all ....

I feel as if I am slowed down:

Nearly all the time ....

Very often ....

Sometimes ....

Not at all ....

I still enjoy the things I used to enjoy:

Definitely as much . . . .

Not quite so much . . . .

Only a little . . . .

Hardly at all . . . .

I get a sort of frightened feeling as if something awful is about to happen:

Very definitely and quite badly . . . .

Yes, but not too badly . . . .

A little, but it doesn't worry me . . . .

Not at all . . . .

I can laugh and see the funny side of things:

As much as I always could . . . .

Not quite so much now . . . .

Definitely not so much now . . . .

Not at all . . . .

I get a sort of frightened feeling like 'butterflies' in the stomach:

Not at all . . . .

Occasionally . . . .

Quite often . . . .

Very often . . . .

I have lost interest in my appearance:

Definitely . . . .

I don't take so much care as I should . .

I may not take quite as much care . . . . .

I take just as much care as ever . . . .

I feel restless as if I have to be on the move:

Very much indeed . . . .

Quite a lot . . . .

Not very much . . . .

Not at all . . . .

I look forward with enjoyment to things:

As much as ever I did . . . .
Rather less than I used to . . . .
Definitely less than I used to . . . . . .
Hardly at all . . . .

I get sudden feelings of panic:

Very often indeed . . . .
Quite often . . . .
Not very often . . . .
Not at all . . . .

I can enjoy a good book or radio or TV programme:

Often . . . .
Sometimes . . . .
Not often . . . .
Very seldom . . . .

Worrying thoughts go through my mind:

A great deal of the time . . . .
A lot of the time . . . .
From time to time but not too often . . . .
Only occasionally . . . .

I feel cheerful:

Not at all . . . .
Not often . . . .
Sometimes . . . .
Most of the time . . . .

I can sit at ease and feel relaxed:

Definitely . . . .
Usually . . . .
Not often . . . .
Not at all . . . .

Reproduced by kind permission of Dr. R. P. Snaith

Appendix IV
Visual analogue scales: patient anxiety

Please read each item and place a cross along each line to indicate how *anxious* you feel about the following:

1. General health

Not at all   Extremely

2. Ability to work

Extremely   Not at all

3. Another heart attack

Extremely   Not at all

4. Relations with spouse

Extremely   Not at all

5. Possible complications

Not at all   Extremely

6. Sexual activity

Extremely   Not at all

7. Leisure activity

Not at all   Extremely

8. The future

Not at all   Extremely

Appendix V
Visual analogue scales: spouse anxiety

Please read each item and place a cross along each line to indicate how *anxious* you feel about the effects of your husband's heart attack on the following:

1. **Your leisure activities**

Extremely   Not at all

2. **Your future**

Not at all   Extremely

3. **Your sexual activities**

Not at all   Extremely

4. **Your general health**

Extremely   Not at all

5. **Your relationship**

Not at all   Extremely

6. **Your husband's ability to work**

Not at all   Extremely

7. **Your husband having another heart attack**

Extremely   Not at all

8. **Possible complications for your husband**

Extremely   Not at all

Appendix VI
Visual analogue scales: patient satisfaction

Please read each item and place a cross along each line to indicate how *satisfied* you feel about the following:

1. General health

Not at all   Extremely

2. Life in general

Extremely   Not at all

3. Care received

Not at all   Extremely

4. Information received

Extremely   Not at all

Appendix VII
Visual analogue scales: spouse satisfaction

Please read each item and place a cross along each line to indicate how *satisfied* you feel about the following:

1. Information received

Extremely   Not at all

2. Care my husband received

Not at all   Extremely

Appendix VIII
Knowledge
questionnaire

Please read the questionnaire carefully and try to answer each question. For questions 1–4 please tick True of False for each statement – there may be more than one true answer!

		True	False
1.	A heart attack is:		
	a) When the heart stops beating	[ ]	[ ]
	b) When an area of heart muscle is damaged by a clot in one of the coronary arteries	[ ]	[ ]
	c) When the heart becomes infected	[ ]	[ ]
2.	Another name for a heart attack is:		
	a) Coronary thrombosis	[ ]	[ ]
	b) Angina	[ ]	[ ]
	c) Myocardial infarction	[ ]	[ ]
3.	The pain associated with a heart attack is generally due to:		
	a) Inflammation of the heart muscle	[ ]	[ ]
	b) Too little oxygen to the heart muscle	[ ]	[ ]
	c) Irritability of the heart muscle	[ ]	[ ]
4.	The cardiac monitor:		
	a) Gives information about the heart's electrical activity	[ ]	[ ]
	b) Helps the heart to beat better	[ ]	[ ]
	c) Warns staff of any changes in the heart's rhythm	[ ]	[ ]

	True	**False**
5. After a heart attack most people will never return to their previous level of fitness	[ ]	[ ]
6. Most people should be fit to return to part-time or light full-time work 6–10 weeks after leaving hospital	[ ]	[ ]

7. List the 3 major 'risk factors' thought to increase the likelihood of a heart attack.

   a)
   b)
   c)

8. How long does it take the damaged heart muscle to heal?

Appendix IX
Activity scale

Please place a cross along the line to indicate your *present* level of general activity compared to the level before your heart attack.

Definitely worse   Definitely better

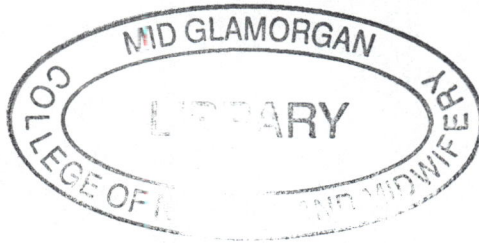

MID GLAMORGAN COLLEGE OF NURSING AND MIDWIFERY LIBRARY

References

Acker J E (1976) Socio-economic factors affected by an in-hospital cardiac rehabilitation program. In: *Psychological Approach to the Rehabilitation of Coronary Patients*, Stockmeier U (ed.) pp.96–100. New York: Springer-Verlag.

Adsett C A and Bruhn J G (1968) Short-term group psychotherapy for post-myocardial infarction patients and their wives. *Canadian Medical Association Journal*, **99**: 577–584.

Aitken R C B (1969) Measurement of feelings using visual analogue scales. *Proceedings of the Royal Society of Medicine*, **62**: 989–993.

Aylard P R, Gooding J H, McKenna P J and Snaith R P (1987) A validation study of three anxiety and depression self-assessment scales. *Journal of Psychosomatic Research*, **31**: 261–268.

Bedsworth J A and Molen M T (1982) Psychological stress in spouses of patients with myocardial infarction. *Heart and Lung*, **11**: 450–456.

Billing E, Lindell B, Sederholm M and Theorell T (1980) Denial, anxiety, and depression following myocardial infarction. *Psychosomatics*, **21**: 639–645.

Blanchard E B and Miller S T (1977) Psychological treatment of cardiovascular disease. *Archives of General Psychiatry*, **34**: 1402–1413.

Bloch A, Maeder J-A and Haissly J-Cl (1975) Sexual problems after myocardial infarction. *American Heart Journal*, **90**: 536–537.

Blumenthal J A and Emery C F (1988) Rehabilitation of patients following myocardial infarction. *Journal of Consulting and Clinical Psychology*, **56**: 374–381.

Bond A and Lader M H (1974) Use of analogue scales in rating subjective feelings. *British Journal of Medical Psychology*, **47**: 211–218.

Bramley P N, Easton A M E, Morley S and Snaith R P (1988) The differentiation of anxiety and depression by rating scales. *Acta Psychiatrica Scandinavica*, **77**: 133–138.

Bulpitt C J (1987) Confidence intervals. *Lancet*, **1**: 494–497.

Byrne D G (1982a) Illness behaviour and psychosocial outcome after a heart attack. *British Journal of Clinical Psychology*, **21**: 145–146.

Byrne D G (1982b) Psychological responses to illness and outcome after survived myocardial infarction: a long term follow-up. *Journal of Psychosomatic Research*, **26**: 105–112.

Byrne D G and Whyte H M (1978) Dimensions of illness behaviour in survivors of myocardial infarction. *Journal of Psychosomatic Research*, **22**: 485–491.

Byrne D G, Whyte H M and Butler K L (1981) Illness behaviour and outcome following survived myocardial infarction: a prospective study. *Journal of Psychosomatic Research*, **25**: 97–107.

Cassem N H and Hackett T P (1971) Psychiatric consultation in a coronary care unit. *Annals of Internal Medicine*, **75**: 9–14.

Cay E L (1982) Psychological problems in patients after a myocardial infarction. *Advances in Cardiology*, **29**: 108–112.

Cay E L, Vetter N J, Philip A E and Dugard P (1972a) Psychological status during recovery from an acute heart attack. *Journal of Psychosomatic Research*, **16**: 425–435.

Cay E L, Vetter N J, Philip A E and Dugard P (1972b) Psychological reactions to a coronary care unit. *Journal of Psychosomatic Research*, **16**: 437–447.

Cay E L, Vetter N J, Philip A E and Dugard P (1973) Return to work after a heart attack. *Journal of Psychosomatic Research*, **17**: 231–243.

Channer K S, James M A, Papouchado M and Rees J R (1985) Anxiety and depression in patients with chest pain referred for exercise testing. *Lancet*, **2**: 820–823.

Channer K S, James M A , Papouchado M and Rees J R (1987) Failure of a negative exercise test to reassure patients with chest pain. *Quarterly Journal of Medicine*, **240**: 315–322.

Cromwell R L, Butterfield E C, Brayfield F M and Curry J J (1977) *Acute Myocardial Infarction: Reaction and Recovery.* St. Louis: C V Mosby.

Croog S H, Levine S and Lurie Z (1968) The heart patient and the recovery process: a review of the literature on social and psychological factors. *Social Science and Medicine*, **2**: 111–164.

Dellipiani A W, Cay E L, Philip A E, Vetter N J, Colling W A, Donaldson R J and McCormack P (1976) Anxiety after a heart attack. *British Heart Journal*, **38**: 752–757.

Doehrman S R (1977) Psycho-social aspects of recovery from coronary heart disease: a review. *Social Science and Medicine*, **11**: 199–218.

Dominian J and Dobson M (1969) Study of patients' psychological attitudes to a coronary care unit. *British Medical Journal*, **4**: 795–798.

Dracup K (1985) A controlled trial of couples group counselling in cardiac rehabilitation. *Journal of Cardiopulmonary Rehabilitation*, **5**: 436–442.

Evans S J W, Mills P and Dawson J (1988) The end of the *p* value? *British Heart Journal*, **60**: 177–180.

Eysenck H J and Eysenck S B G (1975) *Manual of the Eysenck Personality Questionnaire.* London: Hodder and Stoughton.

Fielding R (1979) Behavioural treatment in the rehabilitation of myocardial infarction patients. In: *Research in Psychology and Medicine, Vol. 1*, Oborne D J, Gruneberg M M and Eiser J R (eds.), pp.176–182. London: Academic Press.

Folstein M F and Luria R (1973) Reliability, validity, and clinical application of the visual analogue mood scale. *Psychological Medicine*, **3**: 479–486.

Frank K A, Heller S S and Kornfeld D S (1979) Psychological intervention in coronary heart disease: a review. *General Hospital Psychiatry*, **1**: 18–23.

Gardner M J and Altman D G (1986) Confidence intervals rather than P values: estimation rather than hypothesis testing. *British Medical Journal,* **292**: 746–750.

Garrity T F and Klein R F (1975) Emotional response and clinical severity as early determinants of six-month mortality after myocardial infarction. *Heart and Lung,* **4**: 730–734.

Goldberg D (1985) Identifying psychiatric illness among general medical patients. *British Medical Journal,* **291**: 161–162.

Gottlieb B H (1983) *Social Support Strategies.* Beverly Hills: Sage Publications.

Gruen W (1975) Effects of brief psychotherapy during the hospitalization period on the recovery process in heart attacks. *Journal of Consulting and Clinical Psychology,* **43**: 223–232.

Hackett T P and Cassem N H (1984) Psychologic aspects of rehabilitation after myocardial infarction and coronary artery bypass surgery. In: *Rehabilitation of the Coronary Patient,* 2nd edn. Wenger N K and Hellerstein H K (eds.), pp.437–451. New York: John Wiley and Sons.

Hackett T P, Cassem N H and Wishnie H A (1968) The coronary care unit. An appraisal of its psychological hazards. *New England Journal of Medicine,* **279**:1365–1370.

Hayes M H S and Patterson D G (1921) Experimental development of the graphic rating scale. *Psychological Bulletin,* **18**: 98–99.

Hellerstein H K and Friedman E H (1970) Sexual activity in the post-coronary patient. *Archives of Internal Medicine,* **125**: 987–999.

Hentinen M (1983) Need for instruction and support of the wives of patients with myocardial infarction. *Journal of Advanced Nursing,* **8**: 519–524.

Hinohara S (1970) Psychological aspects in rehabilitation of coronary heart disease. *Scandinavian Journal of Rehabilitation Medicine,* **2**: 53–59.

Horlick L, Cameron R, Firor W, Bhalerao U and Baltzan R (1984) The effects of education and group discussion in the post myocardial infarction patient. *Journal of Psychosomatic Research,* **28**: 485–492.

Ibrahim M A, Feldman J G, Sultz H A, Staiman M G, Young L J and Dean D (1974) Management after myocardial infarction: a controlled trial of the effects of group psychotherapy. *International Journal of Psychiatry in Medicine,* **5**: 253–268.

Jarvis M J, Belcher M, Vesey C and Hutchison D C S (1986) Low cost carbon monoxide monitors in smoking assessment. *Thorax,* **41**: 886–887.

Klein R F, Kliner V A, Zipes D P, Troyer W G and Wallace A G (1968) Transfer from a coronary care unit. Some adverse responses. *Archives of Internal Medicine,* **122**: 104–108.

Langosch W, Seer P, Brodner G, Kallinke D, Kulick B and Heim F (1982) Behaviour therapy with coronary heart disease patients: results of a comparative study. *Journal of Psychosomatic Research,* **26**: 475–484.

Ley P (1988) *Communicating with Patients.* London: Croom Helm.

Lloyd G G and Cawley R H (1978) Psychiatric morbidity in men one week after first acute myocardial infarction. *British Medical Journal,* **2**: 1453–1454.

Lloyd G G and Cawley R H (1982) Psychiatric morbidity after myocardial infarction. *Quarterly Journal of Medicine*, **51**: 33–42.

Lloyd G G and Cawley R H (1983) Distress or illness? A study of psychological symptoms after myocardial infarction. *British Journal of Psychiatry*, **142**: 120–125.

McCormack H M, Horne D J L and Sheather S (1988) Clinical application of visual analogue scales: a critical review. *Psychological Medicine*, **18**: 1007–1019.

Maeland J G and Havik O E (1987) Psychological predictors for return to work after a myocardial infarction. *Journal of Psychosomatic Research*, **31**: 471–481.

Maxwell C (1978) Sensitivity and accuracy of the visual analogue scale: a psychophysical classroom experiment. *British Journal of Clinical Pharmacology*, **6**: 15–24.

Mayberry J F, Kent S V, Jenkins B and Colbourne G (1983) Employment of men after myocardial infarction. *British Medical Journal*, **287**: 1262–1263.

Mayou R (1984) Prediction of emotional and social outcome after a heart attack. *Journal of Psychosomatic Research*, **28**: 17–25.

Mayou R, Williamson B and Foster A (1976) Attitudes and advice after myocardial infarction. *British Medical Journal*, **1**: 1577–1579.

Mayou R, Foster A and Williamson B (1978a) The psychological and social effects of myocardial infarction on wives. *British Medical Journal*, **1**: 699–701.

Mayou R, Foster A and Williamson B (1978b) Psychosocial adjustment in patients one year after myocardial infarction. *Journal of Psychosomatic Research*, **22**: 447–453.

Mayou R, Williamson B and Foster A (1978c) Outcome two months after myocardial infarction. *Journal of Psychosomatic Research*, **22**: 439–445.

Meddis R (1980) Unified analysis of variance by ranks. *British Journal of Mathematical and Statistical Psychology*, **33**: 84–98.

Meddis R (1984) *Statistics Using Ranks. A Unified Approach*. Oxford: Blackwell.

Montgomery S A and Asberg M (1979) A new depression rating scale designed to be sensitive to change. *British Journal of Psychiatry*, **134**: 382–398.

Mumford E, Schlesinger H J and Glass G V (1982) The effects of psychological intervention on recovery from surgery and heart attacks: an analysis of the literature. *American Journal of Public Health*, **72**: 141–151.

Nagle R, Gangola R and Picton-Robinson I (1971) Factors influencing return to work following myocardial infarction. *Lancet*, **2**: 454–456.

Naismith L D, Robinson J F, Shaw G B and MacIntyre M M J (1979) Psychological rehabilitation after myocardial infarction. *British Medical Journal*, **1**: 439–446.

Nichols K A (1984) *Psychological Care in Physical Illness*. London: Croom Helm.

Nichols K A (1985) Psychological care by nurses, paramedical and medical staff: essential developments for the general hospitals. *British Journal of Medical Psychology*, **58**: 231–240.

Norris R M, Brandt P W T, Caughey D E, Lee A J and Scott P J (1969) A new coronary prognostic index. *Lancet*, **1**: 274–278.

Office of Population Censuses and Surveys (1980) *Classification of Occupations*. London: HMSO.

Oldenburg B, Perkins R J and Andrews G (1985) Controlled trial of psychological intervention in myocardial infarction. *Journal of Consulting and Clinical Psychology*, **53**: 852–359.

Padgett D, Mumford E, Hynes M and Carter R (1988) Meta-analysis of the effects of educational and psychosocial interventions on management of diabetes mellitus. *Journal of Clinical Epidemiology*, **41**: 1007–1030.

Peet M (1988) The treatment of anxiety with beta-blocking drugs. *Postgraduate Medical Journal*, **64** (suppl. 2): 45–49.

Perkins R J, Oldenburg B and Andrews G (1986) The role of psychological intervention in the management of patients after myocardial infarction. *Medical Journal of Australia*, **144**: 358–360.

Philip A E, Cay E L, Vetter N J and Stuckey N A (1979) Short-term fluctuations in anxiety in patients with myocardial infarction. *Journal of Psychosomatic Research*, **23**: 277–280.

Philip A E, Cay E L, Stuckey N A and Vetter N J (1981) Multiple predictors and multiple outcomes after myocardial infarction. *Journal of Psychosomatic Research*, **25**: 137–141.

Pocock S J (1983) *Clinical Trials. A Practical Approach*. Chichester: John Wiley and Sons.

Rahe R H, Tuffli C F, Suchor R J and Arthur R J (1973) Group therapy in the outpatient management of post-myocardial infarction patients. *International Journal of Psychiatry in Medicine*, **4**: 77–88.

Rahe R H, Ward H W and Hayes V (1979) Brief group therapy in myocardial infarction rehabilitation: three- to four-year follow-up of a controlled trial. *Psychosomatic Medicine*, **41**: 229–242.

Rampling D J and Williams R A (1977) Evaluation of group processes using visual analogue scales. *Australian and New Zealand Journal of Psychiatry*, **11**: 189–191.

Razin A M (1982) Psychosocial intervention in coronary artery disease: a review. *Psychosomatic Medicine*, **44**: 363–387.

Razin A M (1985) *Helping Cardiac Patients*. San Francisco: Jossey-Bass.

Rose G A, Blackburn H, Gillum R F and Prineas R J (1982) *Cardiovascular Survey Methods*. Geneva: World Health Organisation.

Roviaro S, Holmes D S and Holmsten R D (1984) Influence of a cardiac rehabilitation program on the cardiovascular, psychological, and social functioning of cardiac patients. *Journal of Behavioural Medicine*, **7**: 61–81.

Royal College of Physicians of London (1983) Obesity. *Journal of the Royal College of Physicians of London*, **17**: 3–58.

Sackett D L and Haynes R B (1976) *Compliance with Therapeutic Regimens*. Baltimore: Johns Hopkins University Press.

Schwab J J, Bialow M, Brown J M and Holzer C E (1967) Diagnosing depression in medical inpatients. *Annals of Internal Medicine*, **67**: 695–707.

Silverstone P H (1987) Depression and outcome in acute myocardial infarction. *British Medical Journal*, **294**: 219–220.

Skelton M and Dominian J (1973) Psychological stress in wives of patients with myocardial infarction. *British Medical Journal,* **2**: 101–103.

Snaith R P and Taylor C M (1985) Rating scales for depression and anxiety: a current perspective. *British Journal of Clinical Pharmacology,* **19**: 17S–20S.

Steptoe A (1981) *Psychological Factors in Cardiovascular Disorders.* London: Academic Press.

Stern M J and Cleary P (1982) The national exercise and heart disease project: long-term psychosocial outcome. *Archives of Internal Medicine,* **142**: 1093–1097.

Stern M J and Pascale L (1979) Psychosocial adaptation post-myocardial infarction: the spouse's dilemma. *Journal of Psychosomatic Research,* **23**: 83–87.

Stern M J, Pascale L and McLoone J B (1976) Psychosocial adaptation following an acute myocardial infarction. *Journal of Chronic Diseases,* **29**: 513–526.

Stern M J, Pascale L and Ackerman A (1977) Life adjustment after myocardial infarction. Determining predictive variables. *Archives of Internal Medicine,* **137**: 1680–1685.

Thompson D R and Cordle C J (1988) Support of wives of myocardial infarction patients. *Journal of Advanced Nursing,* **13**: 223–228.

Thompson D R, Cordle C J and Sutton T W (1982) Anxiety in coronary patients. *International Rehabilitation Medicine,* **4**: 161–164.

Thompson D R, Webster R A, Cordle C J and Sutton T W (1987) Specific sources and patterns of anxiety in male patients with first myocardial infarction. *British Journal of Medical Psychology,* **60**: 343–348.

Trelawny-Ross C and Russell O (1986) Social and psychological response to myocardial infarction: multiple determinants of outcome at six months. *Journal of Psychosomatic Research,* **30**: 113–120.

Vetter N J, Cay E L, Philip A E and Strange R C (1977) Anxiety on admission to a coronary care unit. *Journal of Psychosomatic Research,* **21**: 73–78.

Wenger N K (1982) Patient and family education and counselling: a requisite component of cardiac rehabilitation. In: *Controversies in Cardiac Rehabilitation,* Mathes P and Halhuber M J (eds.) pp.108–114. Berlin: Springer-Verlag.

Wiklund I, Sanne H, Vedin A and Wilhelmsson C (1984) Psychosocial outcome one year after a first myocardial infarction. *Journal of Psychosomatic Research,* **28**: 309–321.

Wilson-Barnett J (1984) Interventions to alleviate patients' stress: a review. *Journal of Psychosomatic Research,* **28**: 63–72.

Wilson-Barnett J (1988) Patient teaching or patient counselling? *Journal of Advanced Nursing,* **13**: 215–222.

Winefield H R and Martin C J (1981) Measurement and prediction of recovery after myocardial infarction. *International Journal of Psychiatry in Medicine,* **11**: 145–154.

Wishnie H A, Hackett T P and Cassem N H (1971) Psychological hazards of convalescence following myocardial infarction. *Journal of the American Medical Association,* **215**: 1292–1296.

Wynn A (1967) Unwarranted emotional distress in men with ischaemic heart disease. *Medical Journal of Australia,* **2**: 847–851.

Young D T, Kottke T E, McCall M M and Blume D (1982) A prospective controlled study of in-hospital myocardial infarction rehabilitation. *Journal of Cardiac Rehabilitation,* **2**: 32–40.

Zigmond A S and Snaith R P (1983) The Hospital Anxiety and Depression scale. *Acta Psychiatrica Scandinavica,* **67**: 361–370.

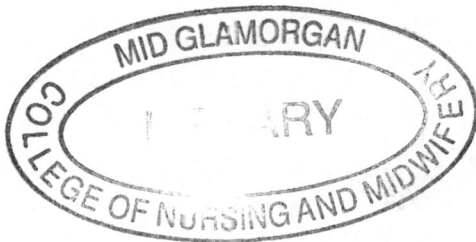

MID GLAMORGAN COLLEGE OF NURSING AND MIDWIFERY LIBRARY